Don't worry and wonder:
Let Dr. Gersh and Dr. Litt
tell you what it's all about.

THE HANDBOOK
OF ADOLESCENCE

Clear and reassuring answers to hundreds of questions about the special problems of young people, including:

Is acne curable?
Can menstrual cramps be prevented?
How tall will you grow?
When should you consider contact lenses?
What are the five stages of breast development?
How can VD be detected?
What are the warning signals of diabetes?
Can exercise solve a weight problem?

An invaluable reference book for both young people and their parents.

Indexed for easy use.

D0988943

THE
Handbook
OF
Adolescence

MARVIN J. GERSH, M.D.
AND IRIS F. LITT, M.D.

A DELL BOOK

Published by
DELL PUBLISHING CO., INC.
1 Dag Hammarskjold Plaza
New York, New York 10017

Reprinted by arrangement with
Stein and Day/Publishers
Printed in the United States of America
First Dell printing—November 1974

Contents

THE
Handbook
OF
Adolescence

Introduction

We would recommend that anyone who wishes to appreciate the biological turbulence, the dissonances, and the hopeful eventual harmony marking the passage through adolescence that our species has always undergone lie down in a quiet room and play at full blast Richard Strauss's *Also Sprach Zarathustra,* which was used as background music for the Dawn of Man sequence in the movie *2001.*

At first one hears some distant drumming—barely perceptible—the first signal that something is going on. It is only vaguely disturbing. Then there are horns rising to a crescendo heralding some inner happening, a volcano bubbling insistently upward, accompanied by a steady martial beat of drums—a reflection of the adolescent's gradual perception of the acquisition of power, a nondirected, unshaped power, but power nevertheless.

The thrust of the music is not unrelenting. Fortissimo alternates with pianissimo. But finally, triumphantly, the horns blare forth, the drums are insistent, and the theme, the process, is complete. Man is born into adulthood.

History bears witness in comments from Aristotle through Shakespeare of the jarring, disturbing nature of adolescence. What makes this particular age different from previous periods is not adolescence itself, but the confused, self-conscious, paralyzed way that we as adults react.

No one can have a solution, if that is the right word to use with regard to contemporary problems of adolescence. There may not be any individual solutions, so powerful are the social forces at work, but we shall attempt to enlighten you about adolescence: what it sets in motion, and what are the dangers, both physical and mental, that are peculiar to its time. If understanding is power, perhaps our exploration will lessen the sense of impotence felt by adolescents and parents alike that have so marked our society.

Adolescence:
Disease or Condition?

The general sense of uneasiness with which we speak about adolescence, and our euphemisms for those undergoing it—teen-agers, young people, the teens—attest to our desire not to face up to it.

Although you might not know it from some contemporary discussions, adolescence is not a disease; it is a human condition. To hark back to our musical metaphor, we can attempt to understand it in broad outline by understanding its theme, the instruments in its orchestra, its conductor, and its audience.

The theme of adolescence is the development, the passage from childhood to adulthood. This transition begins with the first external changes in body hair (the term puberty is derived from the Latin *puber,* meaning hair), and ends—physically, at least—in complete sexual differentiation, male and female, with the capacity for union of these differentiated states in reproduction.

The instruments for this development are the brain, the forebrain, a primordial portion of the brain called the hypothalamus, the pituitary gland or "master gland," and lastly the gonads—the female ovaries and the male testes. At the right time in a child's development the appropriate messages are somehow sent back and forth from the glands to the brain, and puberty begins. We are apparently coded by genetic material in such a way that the onset of puberty is to a large measure predetermined by heredity.

The forebrain, or cerebrum, apparently inhibits the development of adolescence; that is, it keeps the glands in check. As a matter of fact, in some instances when parts of the brain are destroyed by accident or disease, we get a very early onset of adolescence, called sexual precocity.

There is a little-understood, non-secreting gland called the pineal gland, which lies with the brain substance, that is also believed to inhibit the onset of adolescence. If it is diseased, this can also cause sexual precocity.

The hypothalamus is involved too in this regulation. Nerve tracts go from it to the pituitary gland programming the rate of functioning of the various glands.

These instruments do not exist in a vacuum. The vibrancy and health of the sex-hormone-producing organs are influenced by such external factors as nutrition. For example, the onset of adolescence in Japanese girls studied in the 1940s in Japan was significantly later than for Japanese-American girls living in California during the same period of time.

Adolescence now begins significantly earlier than it did, say, one hundred fifty years ago, during the early part of the Industrial Revolution. Its onset is probably now approximately what it was in pre-industrial times in European agricultural communities. This is undoubtedly related to the availability of abundant nutrition.

There are many curious factors affecting the timing of puberty. These are probably initiated through our brain. Whereas light will increase the rate of development of most species, it is the reverse in humans. Blind girls develop significantly earlier than normally sighted girls. We use this as an example to point out the varying and now only shadowily perceived influences on our biological clock.

It is not farfetched to predict that before very long we will be able to control adolescent development, if necessary, without serious disturbance. This will give welcome respite to many a harried parent who has often wished to turn it on and off at will. Then the universal teen-age complaint that grown-ups are always trying to control them will have a biological basis.

CHAPTER ONE

The Development of
the Adolescent

HOW DOES YOUR GARDEN GROW?

Mistress Mary quite contrary
How does your garden grow?
With silver bells and cockle shells
And pretty maids all in a row.

This description of the wonders of female adolescence expresses the sense of awe that we all feel at the transformation from girl to woman. How common it is for someone to see a young lady after a lapse of perhaps a year and remark, after being somewhat shaken, "Why, Mary, the last time I saw you, you were a little girl." This sense of wonder is not confined only to the observer but affects the girl herself, who in some sense is an anxious witness to the rapid glandular developments that change the shape of her body and the nature of her sensations.

If Mary really did know how her garden grew, she would be spared a lot of anxiety. If her parents were knowledgeable about the normal process of adolescence, they could be very helpful to her. Many unnecessary visits to doctors or clinics, in fact the vast majority of them, are prompted by variations in normal development that are misinterpreted by parents and children alike as "gland trouble."

There is considerable difference in the rate and the course of development in each girl, and we feel it would be very helpful for parents and children to know about this.

The first change is fairly subtle. You will probably

say one day, "My, she is getting a figure." This observation is prompted by the fact that her hips are
broadening. This in turn is due to the growth of the
pelvis or hip girdle, the bony part of the birth canal
through which a baby must eventually pass. The usual
female pelvis, in contrast to the male's, has a round,
wide outlet and makes the lower curve of the hour-
glass portion of the figure. Let us hasten to state, however, that there is great variation in the pelvic formation. Not every girl develops broad hips, and this can
be quite normal. The hip or pelvic bony development
generally begins at nine to ten years of age.

The breasts usually start to develop somewhere between eight and thirteen years of age.

Breast development goes through five stages:

1. There is slight elevation of the tissue directly under the nipple.
2. The breast bud stage. The breast itself becomes
   slightly raised to form a mound, and the area
   around the nipple, known as the areola, becomes
   enlarged.
3. Further enlargement occurs in the breast itself
   and then the areola.
4. The nipple, its base, and the areola form a
   mound on the already-mounded breast.
5. The nipple itself projects as the areola flattens
   into the center of the breast.

Remember, the timing of breast development is
very variable. The following are only averages:

First stage—average 10 years, variations 8 to 13
   years
Second stage—average 12 years, variations 8 to 15
   years
Third stage—average 13 years, variations 9 to 15
   years
Fourth stage—average 14 years, variations 11 to 16
   years

Fifth stage—average 16 years, variations 12 to 19 years

You can see from these figures that concern about slow breast development, which is common in our society where the breast is a sex symbol, can be avoided by a knowledge of these variations. This is particularly important to the adolescent who suffers most of the time from severe preoccupation with her body image. A girl slightly slower than her classmates in breast development may receive damage to her self-esteem, via her body image, that will persist long after her development has caught up if this issue is not satisfactorily and factually dealt with when it arises.

A young girl starting breast development is in no danger of not continuing, but there is no guarantee, of course, that the size and shape of her breasts will fit society's current ideal. It is therefore important for parents to de-emphasize whatever the current stereotype perfect figure may be.

There is obviously a good deal less concern about the appearance of pubic hair. It too has an orderly development. It usually roughly keeps pace with breast development, but it may precede or follow breast development and be perfectly normal.

Development of pubic hair proceeds through four stages:

1. Fine, downy hair appears; it is obviously more pronounced in dark-haired children.
2. Hair coarsens, darkens, curls, and spreads out.
3. Hair is now all adult type, coarse and curly.
4. Hair distribution is in the shape of an upside-down triangle; that is, the base is upmost, and the hair borders grow inward and downward to form a V.

First stage—average 13 years, variations 9 to 15 years
Second stage—average 13 years, variations 10 to 16 years

Third stage—average 14 years, variations 11 to 17 years

Fourth stage—average 15 years, variations 12 to 19 years

The appearance of axillary (underarm) hair and general body hair is so variable that it is not a good indicator of development.

One of the best ways to determine when menstrual periods will start is by knowing when the breasts have started to develop. From Stage Two, the budding breast, to the onset of periods, known medically as the menarche, is about two and one-half years, but it may be as little as six months or as long as five years.

We cannot emphasize strongly enough that there is great variation in the rate and the course of development.

Parents frequently worry that seemingly uneven development (such as rapid growth of the breasts without the appearance of genital hair) may indicate that the remainder of the female organs are not developing. There are almost no instances of this occurring. The parent can therefore relax and be reassuring.

It is important to realize that the adolescent naturally has many body-image problems. A parent knowing the normal variations can help in correcting distortions that otherwise could be lifelong. The authors have encountered too many attractive mature women who, stigmatized by an unrealistic adolescent body image, still think of themselves as freakish, as asexual, or as ugly ducklings.

TODAY I AM A MAN

This sentence has been uttered more frequently and with less conviction than perhaps any other. Jewish male children, for instance, undergo, on reaching the age of thirteen, a ceremony (called Bar Mitzvah) which acknowledges that the boy is now officially a man. However, anyone who has heard the high-pitched, faltering voice of a thirteen-year-old will realize the fallacy of relying on chronological age to determine when the passage into maturity is to take place. There is an even more enormous variation in the rate of development in boys than girls. By and large the great majority of boys who get as far as an endocrine clinic, which means they have aroused the concern not only of their parents but indeed of their physicians, are found to be variations of normal.

By far the greatest cause of concern is the delay in the development of boys. Doctors always enjoy a sense of godlike power when they portentously reassure a frightened mother and father that they will most probably be grandparents some day.

How often have we seen a chubby thirteen-year-old with slight broadening of the hips, a beardless face, and the tip of a perfectly normal penis imbedded in fat being accused by his parents of having "gland trouble." We are emphasizing this at this point, and will again, in the hope that we can spare some such child "treatment" with powerful male hormones that will do him no good and may, indeed, do him some harm.

The great variations in development seem to be more cause of concern among boys than among girls. There are several reasons for this. Firstly, because girls mature earlier than boys, boys feel the delay in their development more; they go to classes with girls who are the same chronological age but who could pass for their aunts if not their mothers. Anyone who has been to a junior-high-school dance and seen clusters of attractive young ladies in the same room as shy packs of little boys of the same age will know what I mean.

Secondly, a girl with delays in development can more easily hide it.

Lastly, the variation between boys of the same age is greater. A six-foot, bearded fourteen-year-old getting help from a five-foot, smooth-faced soprano fellow classmate is not an uncommon sight.

Here are the order and variations of normal, not necessarily average (this is an important distinction), growth of a boy.

First stage—the first sign of adolescence in the male is usually the growth of the testes. Average age is 11 years, variations 8 to 14 years.

Second stage—the appearance of fine hair around the penis. Average age is 13 years, variations 10 to 15 years.

Third stage—there then follows a more rapid growth of the penis and testicles. The parents of a perfectly normal 13-year-old with a penis imbedded in fat will at this time obviously become frightened if not reassured. 11 to 15 years.

Fourth stage—there is some enlargement of the area around the nipple as there is in the female. The nipple becomes slightly raised (for the adolescent boy with breast enlargement, see p. 26). There is some spreading out of the pubic hair, forming a triangle with the base uppermost. Average age 14 years, variations 11 to 16 years.

Fifth stage—fine hair on the upper lip, hair in the armpits, and voice change. Average age 14 to 15 years, variations 12 to 17 years.

Sixth stage—beginning of facial hair and possibly some more body hair, not necessarily on the chest but the extremities. There are great personal and hereditary differences. There is some indentation of the hairline at the temples, although this too is variable. At this point the sperm the boy produces are capable of fertilizing an ovum. In other words, he can put someone "in a family way." He should know this, and at the very least he should be told not to rely on Saran Wrap (a common myth in a local high school that may have been responsible for some teen-age marriages). Average age—not for teen-age marriages but for the sixth stage—17 years, variations 14 to 19 years.

CHAPTER TWO

The Adolescent and Body Image

All of us have a mental image, an internal perception, of our physical selves. In essence this is the physical picture that we think we present to other people. The extent to which this image is realistic or distorted influences, to a large extent, our behavior, our relationships with others, our feelings of self-esteem.

Nowhere in the course of human development is the concept of body image more important than in adolescence. No one who has witnessed the preoccupation with mirrors of boys and girls alike can doubt this.

The intensity of this preoccupation is the result of the radical physical change the adolescent undergoes in a relatively short period of time. He really feels he is a stranger in his own body; he is not at home there. This new body, his new home, may appear too large, too unmanageable; one part may appear too small, others too large. His sense of alienation is analogous to the sense of strangeness a New Guinea aborigine might experience if he suddenly found himself in a New York subway.

Anxiety—simply being scared at finding oneself in a new environment—is another inevitable consequence of this rapid change.

There are, of course, realistic concerns that adolescents have about their bodies. These can be alleviated by correct information.

THE SHORT BOY AND DELAYED
ADOLESCENCE

This is one of the most common problems caused by slowness of onset of adolescence. A typical example may be as follows: A fourteen-year-old boy in the eighth grade finds that he is as much as a foot shorter than his classmates, male and female, is beardless, and has a high squeaky voice. Should he not be able to avoid exposing himself in the shower room, his embarrassment and anxiety will be further compounded by the fact that his two-inch penis only recently and sparsely surrounded by fine pubic hairs is the subject of some coarse ridicule by the possessors of six-inch organs, who in loud and deep voices cast unkind reflections on his manhood. More than likely the boy, bitterly confused, anxious, will wind up with some unrealistic concept of what he is really like. It may result, if not dealt with, in permanent distortions that can have an adverse effect on his relationship with women, or even in a more diffuse way on his evaluation of his own efficacy as a person.

Parents may be alerted to this situation when such a boy becomes unduly shy, refuses to go to school dances, or withdraws from social contact with his peers.

There are two approaches. The first is explanation. There may be a family history of delayed adolescence. A careful medical examination is extremely helpful. The physician can determine that the rate of growth is proceeding normally. A blood count, a urinalysis, sometimes an evaluation of thyroid function, will rule out other problems. An X-ray of the wrist to determine bone age, the rate at which various bone centers appear, and when they unite may reveal some slight lag. The important thing is to remember that with this data the boy can be reassured that development *will* take place. Occasionally the physician may choose, for psychological reasons only, to accelerate the adolescent process. By the administration of male hormones or analogues of male hormones, he can speed up the growth of the boy and the development of his secondary sexual characteristics. The beard will appear sooner; so will the pubic hair. There will be a growth spurt, an increase in muscle mass. The ultimate height of the boy, the size of his penis, and the nature of the secondary sexual characteristics are all in the long run usually unchanged; they have just begun to manifest themselves earlier than they would have without medical prodding. The physician and the parents and, most importantly, the boy himself, given the facts, must make the decision to do this together. It is, in fact, not strictly a medical decision, but rather a choice of adolescence now or later. Surely if explanation and reassurance are effective, nothing further should be done.

Sometimes parents do not have insight into their relationships with their boys. Once a parent brought a fourteen-year-old boy in for an evaluation for short stature. He was just under five feet tall, beardless, and strikingly shy. The best way, by the way, of predicting height is to know the height of the parents. In this instance the father was five feet ten inches and had a history of having "shot up" when he was sixteen. After my evaluation the child's mother was assured that he would eventually grow normally, that the only trouble was psychological, and that compassion, preceded, of course, by understanding, could be helpful. The mother stated somewhat defensively that indeed she tried to understand and help him. "I have asked him a thousand times, 'Shorty, why are you so sensitive?' but it doesn't seem to help."

THE TALL GIRL

For every parent concerned that his son is going to be too short, there is a parent concerned that his daughter is going to be too tall. Show me a family where there is a twelve-year-old girl who towers over her fourteen-year-old brother, and I will show you a family with body-image problems. Whenever we examine a girl of ten whose height is on the upper side of normal and whose parent timorously inquires about her height, we have a mental image of what is going on in their minds: It is some eight years hence; Mother and Dad and this six-foot amazon are all unhappily sitting in front of the television set on a Saturday night, and there is no gentleman caller.

A marshaling of the facts might be very helpful. In the first place, girls of twelve are often taller than boys of twelve or fourteen. They mature much earlier—by two years on the average—than boys do.

Secondly, a girl who matures early is likely to be relatively taller at that age. Indeed, girls usually stop growing two years after the onset of menstruation.

Of course, there are six-foot-two-inch girls, but there are also six-foot-four-inch boys. The rather primitive idea that the man must be taller than the girl seems to be disappearing anyway.

Can anything be done, however, about excessive growth in girls? The answer in most instances is Yes.

An unduly tall girl—and size is relative, of course—can be evaluated by a physician. A physician can X-ray the growing ends of the bones, and, if he determines there is still growth to take place, initiate treatment to arrest this growth. By judicious use of female hormones he can cause the growing end of the bone, the epiphysis, to unite with the end shaft of the bone, the metaphysis, at which point growth ceases.

This is not a matter that should be undertaken lightly, and careful observations are necessary.

THE SMALL-PENIS PROBLEM

There are undoubtedly many men, physically normal, whose entire lives have been adversely affected by a sense of sexual inadequacy. In many, the roots of their disturbances can be found in distortion of their sexual image formed in adolescence. A common source of this problem is a misdiagnosis by a physician of the "Froelich syndrome." Many years ago Dr. Froelich described an extremely rare disease of the pituitary (master gland), which results in underdevelopment in the male of his primary (penis and testicles) and his secondary (build, beard, voice, etc.) sexual characteristics. This disease is extremely rare, but unfortunately the term "Froelich syndrome" has been misapplied to multitudes of boys whose ultimate glandular destiny is to be completely normal. Furthermore, many of them have unnecessarily received hormones, which can in themselves, if misapplied and misunderstood, cause psychological damage. The typical misdiagnosed "Froelich" is a moderately obese thirteen-year-old. His fatty tissue is more prominent around somewhat widened hips, and his sense of shyness is in no way helped by a seemingly small penis, inbedded in a mound of fat at the pubic prominence. He looks girlish. If perchance the idea of poor male development has never occurred to him, be assured that some of his friends, tortured by their own self-doubts, will point this out to him to buttress their own shaky feelings of manhood. The parents rarely discuss such a situation with their son until, driven by a gnawing preoccupation, they consult a physician.

Careful examination will usually reveal that the testicles are of normal size, and that the penis is not as small as it appears on first glance, but is simply hidden in the mound of fat.

Such boys and their parents need strong reassurance, probably repeatedly, that the boy will develop masculinity normally. Many endocrinological clinics are filled with such problems. It is important to point out for the sake of reassurance that 90 percent of children referred to endocrine clinics have nothing wrong with them at all in terms of their "glands."

In our age of candor it would not be amiss to assure such a boy that the size of the penis not in erection is no measure of the man, and that furthermore, the size of the penis in any state has nothing to do with the ability to gratify the female.

THE SMALL-BREAST PROBLEM

As we have already pointed out, development, particularly in the female, may be terribly, if not terrifyingly, uneven. Specifically, a girl may have pubic hair, axillary hair, and have begun to menstruate without much breast development. It is unusual, but not abnormal. Such girls do develop breasts by and large (forgive us). A young girl normally developing in other ways can be assured that she will develop breasts. The anxiety of the girl with small breasts is equivalent to the anxiety of the boy with the small penis.

There are, of course, those very rare situations in which there is no breast development, or very little. This is not difficult for the knowledgeable physician to diagnose, and in these instances hormonal therapy is indicated. It is *never* indicated for the girl with uneven development.

BOYS WITH BREASTS

Approximately 50 per cent of adolescent boys have breast tissue (between the fourteenth and fifteenth year). In most cases the breasts merely bud, but in some the breasts may be globular and large. They may also be tender. One side may be more affected than the other. This condition lasts about one to one and one-half years. Although normally this condition occurs naturally, it can be caused by the accidental ingestion of estrogens.

In most instances the only treatment required is reassuring the boy about his masculinity. The breast tissue will go away. In very rare instances, if a boy is suffering severely psychologically, cosmetic surgery is indicated.

Also very rarely, if this condition persists and is associated with small testes, endocrine chromosome studies may have to be done.

The short boy, the tall girl, the small penis, and small breasts are all in the sense realistic problems that can be handled by parent and physician alike by emphasis on the facts.

All adolescents, regardless of their actual physical development, have distortions, dissatisfaction, and consequently, anxieties about their bodies.

It is axiomatic that the more emotionally disturbed the teen-ager, the less sure he is of his body image. Who cannot remember a perfectly stunning young girl, convinced that she is unattractive, bewildered by the attentions shown to her and belittling the poor boys attracted to her—predecessor, perhaps, of a castrating female, a woman so dissatisfied with herself, her own body image, that she feels anyone who could be attracted to one so loathsome must be even more detestable himself.

There are psychiatrists who might state that this woman's self-hate is due to unconscious resentment because she does not have a penis. We believe the latter explanation to be farfetched and the former to be more likely. During this rapid period of physical and psychological change the adolescent is not only more vulnerable to new wounds but more susceptible to the opening up of old ones that have lain quiescent in childhood. Children who always felt inadequate will feel more upset during adolescence. Their sense of discomfort is more than likely to be expressed in terms of dissatisfaction with their bodies. No amount of reassurance—"You are really a very pretty girl"— will help. Feeling inadequate, feeling unloved, they have selectively focused their attention on their bodies. Probably all adolescents feel this way to some degree. The unsureness arising from rapid body change, unfamiliar sensations, new feelings, aggressive and sexual, and awkward movements contribute to a universal manifestation of bodily unease. We do not remember seeing an adolescent girl who did not think she was either too thin or too fat, or in the case of a boy, too thin.

Some of the skinniest adolescent girls we have seen were on diets. There is a possibility that severe distortions of this sort can be the initial signs of a serious disturbance known as *anorexia hervosa* (see page 49).

It is therefore important to meet the situation head-on. If a thin or normal girl is preoccupied with losing weight, the weight problem should be de-emphasized and other areas of her life examined. "You are thin enough" may not be the right approach. Other sources of her unhappiness should be looked into. Her general sense of unattractiveness or some distortions about sexuality can be the cause of this. There have been girls, for example, whose preoccupation with losing weight had its sources in fears that one might become pregnant by eating something. It would be hard in this day of sex education for such fantasy to exist unquestioned, but less exotic misapprehensions often exist.

Many boys feel they are too thin or too weak looking. Some of them try to solve this by endless hours with the barbell. Many adolescent boys in their early years are indeed quite thin, but gain weight rapidly in their later teens. Others may remain thin until middle-aged corpulence sets in. The best single way to predict body build is to look at the parents. The body growth rate and development will often closely follow that of one of the parents, although succeeding generations have been generally bigger and ten pounds heavier than preceding ones since the turn of the century.

THE INFLUENCE OF SOCIETY

We often forget how much pressure the demands of our culture place on the individual. Changes in taste and style can cause real discomfort to an individual whose body type for one reason or another is out of vogue. Compare the plump Rabelaisian female, adipose tissue oozing out of her tightly corseted bodice, wide thighs apart, round arms akimbo, smiling seductively at you from the *Police Gazette,* with the portrait of the heavy lidded bland, drugged countenance of today's model, her swan's neck protruding from an almost linear body, curved at the pubis by an unnatural thrusting back of the trunk.

This change through the years has led to what we call the "Norwegian stringbean syndrome."

Many a girl who reflects her ancestry in a short, somewhat squattish figure and a head encased in curly ringlets, whom you can best envision tending the fire in the camps of Genghis Khan or in the forces of Ivan the Terrible, feels that she must look like the tall, flaxen- and straight-haired, narrow-hipped woman who may or may not have followed Eric the Red to the North American continent.

Hence the large, uncomfortable curlers to straighten naturally curly hair, hence the dieting (see hereditary aspects of obesity, p. 33) to streamline natural voluptuousness; hence the wide belts and tight pants to conceal broad breadth of pelvis.

It is a downright lie that this is the age of everyone doing his own thing. The kind of individuality one finds in fashion and in other areas is that of herds—unthinking, unplanned following—and in this instance stampeding against genetic patterns.

It is hard, of course, to explain to a girl of fourteen that if she really wanted to be a long, thin Norwegian stringbean, she should have chosen different parents. But it seems to us that nothing short of that kind of honest confrontation is likely to be helpful. It is obvious that the electronic media have not been helpful. It is easy to see how the stereotyped image of the ideal body type is engraved on the unformed mind of the average fourteen-year-old, transfixed by the lissome, nubile figure of the latest singing star.

There is a response to the uncertainties and the dissatisfaction of body image that we call the White Swan Syndrome. A young girl, thinking of herself as an ugly goose, becomes withdrawn, spends her time straightening her hair, losing weight, waiting for her braces to be removed. Her fantasy is that in some magical way, with some of her own help, of course, she will wake up one morning and, as in the Hans Christian Andersen fairy tale, find herself a beautiful white swan.

And in some ways, that is almost what happens. As the girl adjusts to her new self, the period of withdrawal ends and she emerges transformed and ready to face the world.

CHAPTER THREE

Weight Problems

MESSAGE FOR AN OBESE TEEN-AGER

Among the more misunderstood minorities of our time, sharing a sense of ignominy with American blacks and Indians, are the approximately 15 million overweight people in the United States, a large proportion of whom suffer from a malady just beginning to be understood, for which they have unjustly been scorned. Our psychological understanding of the obese has been based on a presumed insatiable orality, whose conscious manifestation is gluttony. The net effect has been one of damnation, rendering their task, that of integration into society, all but impossible. Curiously, but understandably, the obese in our country show the same psychological constellation as do other minority groups.

They have a poor self-image, they show tendencies to withdraw, they are plagued with a sense of inferiority and more profoundly with a deep sense of anxiety-producing ugliness.

Like the American black, the obese person has a poorer school record, a lower acceptance rate in college, and a higher unemployment rate.

The history of our attitude toward obesity is interesting and relevant. In the beginning, fatness was considered, as it still is in some parts of the world, a sign of health and prosperity. Images in old *Police Gazettes* of fullsome beauties of their time oozing pink flesh out of their corseted bodices, or the picture of the ample Theodore Roosevelt standing side by side with

William Howard Taft at his inauguration, both proudly and prosperously portly, attest to the time in our recent history when obese people were admired and loved. Think if you will with what derision a 1900 follies queen would be greeted at Atlantic City today. Try to recall one contemporary candidate for major office in this country who was obese. What has happened to all the fat politicians? Styles have changed, and thinness is in. Along with this has come new knowledge that obesity is not a reflection of good health, but on the contrary, is associated with complications that shorten life. At one time pediatricians received complaints that this or that baby was too thin. Now mothers are concerned when an infant of nine months, for example, seems too fat.

As the influence of the grandmother has waned, replaced by that of her daughter, filled with more modern facts and fables, the fat baby has gone out of style. In an attempt to understand obesity, physicians, we must apologetically admit, made two fundamental errors. First, they became hooked on the first law of thermodynamics, namely that matter and energy are in equilibrium and that one is fat simply because one takes in more calories than one expends as energy. It is quite apparent that this notion, applied to the obese, is a destructive oversimplification. Second, physicians assumed that people "overeat" because they have deep psychological problems. In our so-called understanding of obesity we had merely switched labels. A fat person was no longer a victim of his own avariciousness: he had some profound unconscious problem. As one obese teen-age girl said recently, "It is not bad enough that I am fat, I am also accused [her words] of having a deep personality problem. I am unhappy because I am fat, I am not fat because I am unhappy." Her observation was, it seems, quite accurate. She nows carries a double burden.

There can no longer be much doubt that there are in those with resistant, lifelong obesity some as yet incompletely understood abnormalities in energy metabolism. Let us hasten to emphasize, however, that the usually held idea that fat people suffer from some sort of "gland trouble" is false. The explanation lies in some newly elucidated formulation of the ability or the inability to convert fat into energy. Since obesity is only a symptom and not a disease, there are, of course, many causes and situations under which it occurs.

In general there are several types of overweight problems that one need not worry about.

In the first place many children put on weight around ten or eleven years of age and lose it by fifteen or sixteen. We can recall many plump eleven-year-old boys, with a disturbing collection of fat around their hips, giving them a feminine appearance, resulting often in a misdiagnosis of "Froelich Syndrome" (see page 25), who turn out to be wiry, muscular seventeen-year-olds. Equally apparent have been chubby eleven-year-old girls, their recently added weight the hallmark of the approach of adolescence, who readily acquired at sixteen the socially acceptable "Norwegian stringbean" look.

There are people who temporarily put on weight as a reaction to emotional trauma, but they are not really the hard-core predetermined obese that we extend our compassion to. In short, there is a fair amount of transient obesity, which passes for the real thing.

The cause of true obesity is genetic. The truly obese, if not born fat, are born with a marked tendency in that direction. It is well-established but largely unknown that real obesity is a hereditary affair. We owe thanks for this information to Jean Mayer of Harvard, who has taught us so much about the problem in many ways.

Dr. Mayer has shown in his studies that if both parents are normal, there is an 8 or 9 percent chance of the children being fat; if one parent is obese, there is a 40 percent chance of the children being fat; and if both parents are obese, the chances are 80 percent that the children will be obese.

But, you say, that is simply a matter of learning. The parents overeat; the children overeat. The answer to that one is that these statistics do not hold for adopted children. On the contrary, we have observed, as others have, that when slim adoptive parents adopt children from obese natural parents, the children follow the obese patterns of their natural parents.

To say that obesity is hereditary and leave it at that is to oversimplify and to leave a sense of resignation, neither of which we intend to do. We are hopeful that by explaining what is really going on we can relieve the sense of secret shame that many overweight teenagers are burdened with. Furthermore, we would like to show them what they are really up against so that they can proudly accept the challenge to "go against the grain."

Much of what we are about to say is not completely understood, but it is beyond reasonable doubt that the energy metabolism of the large majority of obese people differs from that of people whose weight is normal.

An obese person is a fat person. His problem is not overweight, but overaccumulation of fat. The best way to determine obesity is to measure the skin folds to see how much fat they contain. There are standards for this, but the method is a little impractical for home use.

In actuality we would say that someone is obese if his weight is more than 20 percent over the standard listed on the tables on pages 36-37. Unless one is unusually muscular, this formula will hold.

Perhaps some biochemistry would be pertinent at this point. Fat in the body is largely derived from ingested carbohydrates and sweets, which if not used as energy are converted by the body into fat.

Ingested fats are also converted and stored as human fat. Protein foods (meats and eggs, for example), if eaten in relative excess, can be stored as fat. This latter is not well known, and excess protein forms the basis of some pretty intolerable diets that may temporarily result in weight loss, but do not really solve the problem.

Fats are stored in the body as substances known as triglycerides. Under ordinary circumstances, when there are no longer any carbohydrates available for energy, these triglycerides are burned as a source of energy. There are certain enzymes that figure in this conversion. Furthermore, insulin, the level of which is usually elevated in the obese person, may cause carbohydrates to be used either as a source of energy for the muscles or cause them to be converted to fat.

Let us assume that in the fat person—there are animal models that bear out this assumption—the triglycerides are for some reason not converted or burned as a source of energy, and that furthermore, the available carbohydrate is mostly converted to fat. What is the result? The poor obese person does not get the energy he needs, tends to move about less, accumulates more fat from inactivity, and is caught in a vicious circular pattern that he cannot break out of.

To use a more familiar analogy, it is as if a car were repeatedly filled with gas, but because of defective spark plugs (enzymes), barely inched along as the gas tank overflowed. But a human being has will, motivation, and sensitivity, and so he struggles and suffers to overcome the defective spark plugs nature fitted him with.

The fat teen-ager is in a state of hypometabolism (not to be confused with the more familiar "low metabolism" due to low thyroid). It is important to emphasize that the obese teen-ager is not suffering from "gland trouble," nor on the other hand does he have a deep-seated personality problem. The inefficacy of conventional psychotherapy is witness to that, and the effectiveness, sometimes, of groups in helping is by no means evidence that obesity is an emotional disorder.

Quade, a Swedish physician, in what we regard as a definitive study of obese children showed that they had no more basic psychological problems than their non-obese peers, but they did have some superim-

Height-Weight-Age Table for Boys of School Age[1]

(Weight is expressed in pounds)

ht. ins.	5 yrs.	6 yrs.	7 yrs.	8 yrs.	9 yrs.	10 yrs.	11 yrs.	12 yrs.	13 yrs.	14 yrs.	15 yrs.	16 yrs.	17 yrs.	18 yrs.	19 yrs.	ht. ins.
38	34	34														38
39	35	35														39
40	36	36														40
41	38	38	38													41
42	39	39	39	39												42
43	41	41	41	41												43
44	44	44	44	44												44
45	46	46	46	46	46											45
46	47	48	48	48	48											46
47	49	50	50	50	50	50										47
48		52	53	53	53	53										48
49		55	55	55	55	55	55									49
50		57	58	58	58	58	58	58								50
51			61	61	61	61	61	61								51
52			63	64	64	64	64	64	64							52
53			66	67	67	67	67	68	68							53
54				70	70	70	70	71	71	72						54
55				72	72	73	73	74	74	74						55
56				75	76	77	77	77	78	78	80					56
57					79	80	81	81		83	83					57
58						83	84	84	85	85	86	87				58
59						87	88	89	89	90	90	90				59
60						91	92	92	93	94	95	96				60
61							95	96	97	99	100	103	106			61
62							100	101	102	103	104	107	111	116		62
63							105	106	107	108	110	113	118	123	127	63
64								109	111	113	115	117	121	126	130	64
65								114	117	118	120	122	127	131	134	65
66									119	122	125	128	132	136	139	66
67									124	128	130	134	136	139	142	67
68										134	134	137	141	143	147	68
69										137	139	143	146	149	152	69
70										143	144	145	148	151	155	70
71										148	150	151	152	154	159	71
72											153	155	156	158	163	72
73											157	160	162	164	167	73
74											160	164	168	170	171	74

The following percentages of net weight have been added for clothing (shoes and sweaters not included): 35 to 64 pounds: 3.5 per cent; 64 pounds and over: 2.0 per cent.

[1]From material prepared by Bird T. Baldwin, Ph.D., Iowa Child Welfare Research Station, State University of Iowa, and Thomas D. Wood, M.D., Columbia University, New York.

Height–Weight–Age Table for Girls of School Age[1]

(Weight is expressed in pounds)

ht. ins.	5 yrs.	6 yrs.	7 yrs.	8 yrs.	9 yrs.	10 yrs.	11 yrs.	12 yrs.	13 yrs.	14 yrs.	15 yrs.	16 yrs.	17 yrs.	18 yrs.	ht. ins.
38	33	33													38
39	34	34													39
40	36	36	36												40
41	37	37	37												41
42	39	39	39												42
43	41	41	41	41											43
44	42	42	42	42											44
45	45	45	45	45	45										45
46	47	47	47	48	48										46
47	49	50	50	50	50	50									47
48		52	52	52	52	53									48
49		54	54	55	55	56	56								49
50		56	56	57	58	59	61	62							50
51			59	60	61	61	63	65							51
52			63	64	64	64	65	67							52
53			66	67	67	68	68	69	71						53
54				69	70	70	71	71	73						54
55				72	74	74	74	75	77	78					55
56					76	78	78	79	81	83					56
57					80	82	82	82	84	88	92				57
58						84	86	86	88	93	96	101			58
59						87	90	90	92	96	100	103	104		59
60						91	95	95	97	101	105	108	109	111	60
61							99	100	101	105	108	112	113	116	61
62							104	105	106	109	113	115	117	118	62
63								110	110	112	116	117	119	120	63
64								114	115	117	119	120	122	123	64
65								118	120	121	122	123	125	126	65
66									124	124	125	128	129	130	66
67									128	130	131	133	133	135	67
68									131	133	135	136	138	138	68
69										135	137	138	140	142	69
70										136	138	140	142	144	70
71										138	140	142	144	145	71

The following percentages of net weight have been added for clothing (shoes and sweaters not included): 35 to 65 pounds: 3.0 per cent; 66 to 82 pounds: 2.5 per cent; 83 pounds and over: 2 per cent.

[1] From material prepared by Bird T. Baldwin, Ph.D., Iowa Child Welfare Research Station, State University of Iowa, and Thomas D. Wood, M.D., Columbia University, New York.

posed problems because they were obese. Countless numbers of overweight teen-agers have been made to suffer unnecessarily in the name of "psychological" understanding.

Our purpose in writing this is not to ask you, if you are overweight, to resignedly accept your genetic fate, but to give you an understanding of what you are really up against. In that way you can attack the problem with a sense of dignified challenge.

HOW TO LOSE WEIGHT IN THE LONG RUN

You are, if you are to be successful in controlling your malady, going to have to go against the grain. Your spark plugs are defective, and the engine does not start properly or run smoothly, but it is our experience that once the motor gets going it is not half bad. The trick is to get started.

The average obese teen-ager shuns exercise. He quite correctly, it appears, perceives that his machine is hard to get going. He must force himself. Ask an old plump jogger. The first quarter-mile is the toughest, and it never gets easier.

Regular exercise has not been emphasized enough. For example, if you were to walk a mile a day, although you could barely note any daily changes on your scale, you would be at least ten pounds lighter in a year.

Running about ten minutes a day is equivalent to running about a mile a day. Just remember, it is particularly difficult for *you* to get started, but once you get going it is not so bad. Notice we did not say it is pleasant. It need not be fun, but that is life. If you are shy about performing outside, there are inexpensive joggers that you can run on at home that are easy on the knees and on the foundation.

We started off with exercise because we think too little attention has been paid to that aspect of weight loss, but, of course, food intake is important. There are some lucky people whose food intake is regulated by their needs. Their appetites turn off when their metabolic needs are met. If this mechanism is out of control, as it is in many people, and a small error favoring input over output is made, obesity results. So the overweight teen-ager cannot rely on a natural turn-off switch. He must watch his diet. On the one hand, a small error in intake results in overweight; but on the other hand, a steady reduction in intake can result in weight reduction.

Here is how it works. One pound of stored fat equals 3500 calories. To lose this pound, you simply—but persistently—must eat 350 calories a day less than you expend for 10 days. If you keep this up, you can lose 35 pounds in a year. If, as we have seen, you also walk one mile a day, or run ten minutes a day, you can lose 45 pounds in a year.

The following is approximately the number of calories you require for maintenance:

100 pounds	2000 calories
110 pounds	2200 calories
120 pounds	2400 calories
130 pounds	2600 calories
140 pounds	2800 calories
150 pounds	3000 calories
160 pounds	3200 calories
170 pounds	3400 calories
180 pounds	3600 calories

If you are moderately active, taking in the numbers of calories in the right-hand column will maintain your weight at about the level indicated in the left-hand column. But let us say that, as determined by the chart on pages 36-37, you are overweight. You weigh 140 pounds, and you should weigh 120 pounds. All you need to do is reduce your intake by 400 calories a day, and in about six months you will have lost the weight. Figure it out for yourself: 20 pounds times 3500 calories is 70,000 calories, that amount you need to expend. Reducing calories by 400 per day for 170 days, nearly six months, will do it. But, you say, 400 calories is a lot. Not so. It represents a reduction in your daily intake of one piece of pie plus one and a half pieces of toast—or one dessert and a glass of whole milk—or one candy bar and one hamburger roll—in other words, lots of the junk foods that we eat in small amounts anyway.

You can lose weight in the long run, or even in the short run for that matter. The following is a list of exercises with which you will expend the indicated amounts of energy.

Walking briskly (3 miles per hour)	½ hour/120 cal.
Running, horizontal (6 miles per hour)	10 min./160 cal.
Swimming, breast stroke or crawl, average swimmer	10 min./200 cal.
Skiing, snow horizontal	½ hour/240 cal.
Rowing	½ hour/150 cal.
Ice Skating	½ hour/240 cal.
Bicycling (9 miles per hour)	½ hour/150 cal.
Making Beds	½ hour/210 cal.

The results of exercise are not immediately apparent, but regular daily exercise makes an enormous difference. For example, if you walked briskly for one half hour each day you would expend 120 calories. Multiply this by 365 days and you have 43,800 calories. This divided by 3500 (calories per 1 pound body fat) equals 12½ pounds. You would weigh 12½ pounds less at the end of a year. Running for 10 minutes each day would result in a loss of 160 calories per day, or an almost 17-pound weight loss at the end of a year.

A simple way to figure it out is to take the calories expended each day and divide by 10. The answer approximately equals the pounds of fat burned and lost each year with daily exercises. For example, bicycling one-half hour at 9 miles per hour per day would result in burning 15 pounds of fat in one year. A program of daily exercise can control and then prevent obesity in later years.

The following are some prepared diets. An effective diet should taste good and be appealing.

DIETS

1003 calories

calories

BREAKFAST

4 stewed prunes (without sugar)	73
1 med. English muffin (without butter)	125
1 tbsp. jam	60
Coffee or tea (without sugar or milk)	0
	258

LUNCH

3 oz. broiled ground steak	147
6 large fresh mushrooms, broiled	15
1 cup cooked waxed beans	27
Coffee or tea (without sugar or milk)	0
	189

MIDDAY SNACK

¼ cantaloupe	19
Coffee or tea (without sugar or milk)	0
	19

DINNER

5 oz. broiled halibut steak	259
½ cup cooked broccoli	22
1 med. baked potato (without butter)	97
1 med. banana	85
Coffee or tea (without sugar or milk)	0
	463

EVENING SNACK

2 Ritz crackers	30
½ cup skimmed milk	44
	74

986 calories

calories

BREAKFAST

½ med. sliced orange	35
1 soft-boiled egg	77
1 slice toast (without butter)	55
½ cup skimmed milk	44
Coffee or tea (without sugar or milk)	0
	211

LUNCH

3 slices broiled bacon	144
2 slices tomato	15
1 slice whole-wheat toast (without butter)	40
½ cup skimmed milk	44
Coffee or tea (without sugar or milk)	0
	243

MIDDAY SNACK

1 cup bouillon	10
2 Ritz crackers	30
	40

DINNER

6 oz. lean roast beef	220
½ cup rice	85
Lettuce with garlic and 2 tsp. wine vinegar	16
1 sliced tomato	25
½ cup sliced fresh pineapple	32
	378

EVENING SNACK

2 graham crackers	70
½ cup skimmed milk	44
	114

1015 calories

calories

BREAKFAST

½ cup orange juice	53
1 med. egg, scrambled in 1 tsp. butter	77
1 slice white toast (without butter)	75
Coffee or tea (without sugar or milk)	0
	205

LUNCH

1 cup diced fresh pineapple	75
5 tbsp. creamed cottage cheese	80
4 Ritz crackers	60
Coffee or tea (without sugar or milk)	0
	215

MIDDAY SNACK

1 med. fresh pear	60
Coffee or tea (without sugar or milk)	0
	60

DINNER

4 oz. broiled sirloin steak	250
6 lettuce leaves	18
1 sliced med. tomato	25
12 slices cucumbers	10
½ cup fresh fruit salad	68
2 vanilla wafer cookies	50
Coffee or tea (without sugar or milk)	0
	421

EVENING SNACK

2 graham crackers	70
½ cup skimmed milk	44
	114

1092 calories

calories

BREAKFAST

½ grapefruit	48
1 slice whole-wheat toast	55
with 1 tsp. butter	34
1 tsp. strawberry jam	19
½ cup skimmed milk	44
Coffee or tea (without sugar or milk)	0
	200

LUNCH

3 oz. broiled ground steak	147
½ English muffin (without butter)	63
1 tsp. relish	5
½ cup fresh strawberries	27
½ cup skimmed milk	44
	286

MIDDAY SNACK

1 cup tomato juice	50
2 Ritz crackers	30
	80

DINNER

¼ lb. broiled fillet of sole	220
1 med. boiled potato	97
1 cup cooked spinach	45
⅔ cup diced cantaloupe	20
Coffee or tea (without sugar or milk)	0
	382

EVENING SNACK

2 graham crackers	70
½ cup skimmed milk	44
	144

1070 calories

calories

BREAKFAST

½ cantaloupe	35
¾ cup puffed wheat (unsweetened)	33
1 tsp. sugar	16
⅓ cup skimmed milk	29
Coffee or tea (without sugar or milk)	0
	113

LUNCH

2-egg omelet	154
cooked in 1 tsp. butter	50
1 slice toast (without butter)	60
Coffee or tea (without sugar or milk)	0
	264

MIDDAY SNACK

½ cup tomato juice	25
2 Ritz crackers	30
	55

DINNER

4 oz. broiled flank steak	360
6 asparagus spears	21
½ med. baked potato	49
2 slices tomato	15
2 canned pear halves	79
	524

EVENING SNACK

2 graham crackers	70
½ cup skimmed milk	44
	114

1121 calories

calories

BREAKFAST

½ cup orange juice	53
1 med. soft-boiled egg	77
1 slice whole wheat toast (without butter)	55
Coffee or tea (without sugar or milk)	0
	185

LUNCH

1 slice baked ham	100
½ slice swiss cheese	50
1 slice light rye bread (without butter)	55
½ glass skimmed milk	44
½ cup diced cantaloupe	15
Coffee or tea (without sugar or milk)	0
	264

MIDDAY SNACK

1 apple	70
1 cup bouillon	10
	80

DINNER

5 oz. lean roasted leg of lamb	263
1 med. roasted potato	118
½ cup cooked broccoli	22
1 cup diced pineapple	75
Coffee or tea (without sugar or milk)	0
	478

EVENING SNACK

2 graham crackers	70
½ cup skimmed milk	44
	114

1169 calories

calories

BREAKFAST

½ cup orange juice	53
1 soft-boiled egg	75
1 slice toast	75
with 1 pat butter	50
1 glass skimmed milk	44
Coffee or tea (without sugar or milk)	0
	297

LUNCH

5 large shrimps	50
6 large leaves lettuce	18
2 slices tomato	15
6 asparagus spears	21
1 slice whole-wheat bread (without butter)	55
½ cup skimmed milk	44
Coffee or tea (without sugar or milk)	0
	203

MIDDAY SNACK

½ cup strawberries	27
with 2 tbsp. skimmed milk	11
	38

DINNER

6 oz. broiled chicken	230
1 cup cooked green beans	25
1 cup cooked summer squash	34
½ cup apple sauce	150
½ cup fruit jello	78
Coffee or tea (without sugar or milk)	0
	517

EVENING SNACK

2 graham crackers	70
½ cup skimmed milk	44
	114

SUMMARY ON A NOTE OF OPTIMISM

If you are obese, it does not mean that you have a deep personality problem. You have enough to contend with without that erroneous assumption. You have inherited bad spark plugs (enzymes), which makes it tough for you to convert fat into energy. You do, however, have a social problem. Society is prejudiced against you as it is against other minorities. But you do not have to believe the propaganda. Although the long Norwegian-stringbean look is now in vogue, it was not always so. There are many men, for example, who find ample flesh and a fullsome figure exciting, provided that the flesh is not tortured by trying to pass for "thin." Plan a diet. Eat three meals a day. Do not try a crash or fad diet. You must learn to live and deal with your problem unless and until medical science can correct it for you.

Go against the grain. It is not easy for you to get started exercising. Time and motion studies show that even while you are playing tennis you move around 80 percent less than your energetic thin counterpart. Running, bicycling, walking, even though it is hard to get going are tremendously important. (We would eliminate the school bus and build safe sidewalks for kids to walk on if we were on the planning board.) Whether you become as thin as you want to be or not, above all be compassionate with yourself.

ANOREXIA NERVOSA

In our mad pursuit of the currently fashionable state of thinness, we may—and how this occurs is by no means clear—inadvertently cause problems with most serious if not fatal consequences.

Anorexia nervosa was clinically delineated by the English physician Gull, who first wrote of it in 1867. Its absence in ancient, less fashion-conscious times and places may not be accidental. Since its onset is usually insidious, and since to be treated it must be detected early, a typical description is now in order. Our subject is a fourteen-year-old girl (practically all victims are girls) who may decide one day that she is fat. She may or may not be obese, but—and this is crucial—her image of herself is somewhat distorted. She goes on a diet, usually a fairly strict one. She may exist on coffee, toast, or broth for days at a time. She may, however, in the early stages of this disease punctuate her state of almost total food deprivation with food binges. She may eat a quart of ice cream at one sitting and then not eat at all, or eat practically nothing, for the next week. She may in the beginning be overactive. She may lose some weight. She may constantly look at herself in the mirror from all angles and never express satisfaction about her weight loss. As the process proceeds, she will lose her desire for food and stop complaining of hunger. She may, if she thinks she has overeaten, induce vomiting. She may take cathartics or insist on enemas to eliminate food products. In short she has become a fanatic in food avoidance.

If nothing is done to interrupt this morbid process, she will continue to lose weight until the point of emaciation. Carried to this extreme, she will follow a path from emaciation to marked fatigue, complaints of coldness, lack of energy, loss of menstrual periods, and wasting until death.

We cannot overemphasize the gravity of this situation.

There have been many psychoanalytic theories as to the cause of *anorexia nervosa*. One theory holds that the patient with *anorexia nervosa* has a strong oral sadistic compulsion, a tremendous desire to bite or tear with the teeth, and the disease is a result of the repression of that drive, resulting in starvation. Another theory holds that by not eating, the adolescent can destroy the hated incorporated mother within her.

Theories or no, the efficacy of deep psychoanalytic treatment is not proven.

Perhaps the clearest formulation of this problem is

the one put forth most recently. Adolescent girls with *anorexia nervosa* have the conscious or unconscious goal of achieving mastery and independence of their bodies, their form, and its functions. They have severe disturbances of body image so that they are unable to evaluate their own body proportions correctly. They never, even when severely emaciated, regard themselves as thin.

They fail to respond, after a while, to their own bodily needs via stimuli from their intestinal tracts. They do not, after a while, experience hunger. They complain of a lack of feeling for anything and do not recognize their own emotional needs. They feel completely ineffective and powerless as human beings.

We want at this point to contrast them with the ordinary, perhaps a trifle hysterical, weight-conscious adolescent. She certainly complains of hunger. She certainly complains of weakness. She can recognize that she has lost weight.

What can parents or peers do? First, they can recognize the situation. They can try to de-emphasize the adolescent's dissatisfaction with her body image. Should this fail, and should they see the teen-ager's relentless pursuit of weight loss continuing to an irrational point, then they should insist that she see a doctor.

What will the doctor do? There are many approaches. His first job, of course, will be to rule out some known physical cause. The disease that *anorexia nervosa* is most likely to be confused with is a form of gland trouble called hypopituitarism in which the master gland, the pituitary, fails to stimulate the thyroid gland and the adrenal and sexual glands. This is not a difficult distinction for the physician to make.

Having ascertained what the problem is, he may insist on hospitalization. He may have to feed the patient via a stomach pump or intravenously, or both. At the same time, depending on his persuasion, he will engage her in conversation. He will, of course, be non-judgmental. He will try to sort out the conflicts and bring to light the fantasies, if they are present, that are driving the patient toward self-destruction. He will, and this is most important, try to make the patient once again aware of her own impulses, impulses that she may have lost from malnutrition, make her aware of her own feelings, and establish a relationship of trust.

At the same time, the side effects—the anemia, the lack of vitamins, the undernutrition—must all be corrected.

As with many of the other illnesses that afflict man, the exact nature of *anorexia nervosa* and its cause, if there be a single one, await further investigation. It can usually be treated and death prevented, but it is such a grave problem that death still occasionally occurs.

CHAPTER FOUR

The Anatomy of a Female

BASIC GYNECOLOGIC ANATOMY

Down with diagrams of female anatomy in cross-section that require the eye of a butcher to interpret! What teen-agers need is a functional understanding of their anatomy. "Which is the opening for urine?" and "Where is this tampon supposed to fit?" These are some of the questions that need answering. The following is offered as a mirror view of the female external genitalia for the purpose of answering these and other questions:

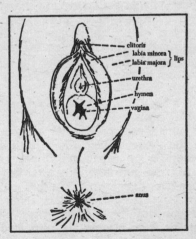

Notice that the lips, or protective covering, are actually made up of two components, the labia majora (covered with hair after puberty) and the inner, moist labia minora. This is important from the point of "good feminine hygiene" (a term that is always mentioned, but rarely explained), for normal vaginal secretions can remain between the minor and major lips and eventually cause an odor if careful attention is not paid to cleaning between them. Douching is never needed for this purpose and may actually be harmful because it can change the bacterial flora and remove protective secretions from the genital canal.

The clitoris is the female counterpart of the penis. The urethra is the tube that leads from the urinary bladder and is entirely separate from the vagina. The hymen or "maidenhead" is a thick membrane that stretches across the vaginal opening. Contrary to popular opinion, it is not an intact barrier, but has an opening of variable size in its center portion. Were this not the case, menstrual flow would have no means of exit from the vaginal canal, and surgical intervention would be necessary. This opening is stretched during intercourse, and the hymenal membrane eventually exists only as a ring around the vagina. In rare instances the hymen may be so tough as to resist stretching and render intercourse painful. A routine gynecologic examination prior to marriage will detect this as well as other minor variations of anatomy that can usually be corrected before they become the source of marital anxiety.

"But if I have a gynecologic examination I will no longer be a virgin." This is a widely held misconception. As mentioned previously, an opening already exists in the hymen which easily admits the doctor's lubricated finger or instruments (speculum) made especially for the purpose of examining young girls. Remember also that a vaginal examination is not always part of the evaluation for some female complaints. Frequently the doctor can get all the information he needs from placing his lubricated finger in the rectum (much like the sensation of having your temperature taken) and feeling the abdomen with his other hand. A young girl undergoing her first gynecologic examination should try to relax. Although this is not easy to do, it really helps, for tensing constricts the vaginal or rectal opening and makes the examination uncomfortable.

Along these same lines, mothers are frequently concerned lest using a sanitary tampon will interfere with their daughters' virginity. The same answer holds. The hymenal opening is sufficient to permit insertion of a tampon. While using tampons is esthetically more satisfying to most girls, it is not without drawbacks. "Out of sight, out of mind" is a potential problem, for if tampons are not changed frequently, the stagnant menstrual flow can provide a good medium for growth of bacteria and produce infection.

DISORDERS OF THE EXTERNAL GENITALIA

The external genitalia are composed basically of skin and mucous membranes, as is the rest of the body. They are therefore subject to many of the same disorders as these tissues elsewhere. If this fact is kept in mind, the appearance of a lesion on the genitalia will not be greeted with alarm.

Most people would not worry about a wart on the hand, but find a bump that looks like a wart near the vagina, and it becomes a medical emergency. The usual genital wart is called *condyloma accuminata* and is caused by a virus, just as is the one on the hand. Treatment usually consists of touching the lesion with a liquid (podophilin) for two or three treatments. The bumps caused by syphilis are much rarer and can be easily distinguished from this common wart by a physician.

Just as a "cold sore" can appear on the lip or in the mouth, the same kind of lesion can occasionally appear on the mucous membranes of the vagina. Both are caused by a virus (*herpes simplex*) and can be quite painful. A sitz bath (sitting in a waist-high tub of hot water for about half an hour) can provide temporary relief from discomfort. Because of some pre-liminary findings that there may be a connection be-tween this virus and cancer in later life, it is wise for the girl afflicted with these sores in the genital area to have a yearly Pap smear taken. It is probably a good idea anyway for all girls to get into a routine of hav-ing a yearly gynecologic checkup even before they reach adulthood.

GYNECOLOGICAL PROBLEMS

The Waiting is Unbearable

Curious, isn't it, that all "female" conditions have in their names the word "men." Actually, this is based on the Greek word for month, rather than the male of the species. The prefix and suffix are added to this root to describe a particular aberration of monthly bleeding. Hence, amenorrhea means absence of month-ly bleeding; dysmenorrhea refers to painful menses; menorrhagia translates literally as bursting forth of menses or more practically, excessive bleeding; oligo-menorrhea means a decrease in the frequency of men-ses; menarche, the age that menstrual function begins; and menopause, the age at which menstrual function ceases.

"I am fourteen and haven't gotten my period. All my friends got theirs more than a year ago." This worry is one of the most frequent causes for an ado-lescent female's visit to a doctor. Underlying her statement is an unspoken fear about her feminity, her future reproductive capacity, and, above all, her de-sire not to be different from her friends. Much of young girls' time together is spent comparing notes about their menses: about cramps and remedies for it; instructions on how to insert tampons; and exchang-ing anecdotes about embarrassing moments when a period came unexpectedly. A girl who has not yet menstruated is left out of this conversation.

There is a definite trend to earlier menarche. On the average menarche occurs today in the United States nine months earlier than ten years ago. Our recent survey of girls in the New York City area indicates that the average age for menarche is now twelve. Remember, however, that this is an average, and as such, it represents the numerical average of the girl who menstruates at eight and the one who starts at sixteen. The girl who menstruates at twelve is no more "normal" than the one who starts at eight or sixteen. She simply has more friends who begin at the same age as she. In other words, "average" is not the same as "normal."

There really is no perfect way for predicting when any individual will menstruate. Thus far, everything short of which shoe a girl puts on first each morning has been shown to influence menarche. Nutrition, rural versus urban living, socio-economic status, chronic illness, blindness, and the amount of maternal loving in childhood have all been implicated.

If small bones called sesamoids have appeared in the thumb, a girl will menstruate within two years, according to one X-ray specialist. Simpler than taking X-rays, however, is asking the mother when she first menstruated. Assuming her good health at the time, it is reasonable to expect that the daughter will begin to menstruate within one year of the time that her mother did.

When a physician is faced with the teen-ager who is concerned about possible amenorrhea, he will inquire about her general health, about symptoms of various endocrine disorders, about the time of appearance of secondary sexual characteristics, about recurrent lower abdominal pain, and even about the health of great-aunts and -uncles. Much of this may seem superfluous, but really isn't. The physical examination that follows will include attention to details of hair, skin, nails, and even ankle and knee jerks, which again may prompt the girl to ask if the doctor remembers that it was her menses she was concerned with. A pelvic examination always takes place in order to be sure that the uterus is normal and that an imperforate hymen is not the cause of absent menses. Depending on what is found on examination, certain blood tests may be in order. Through these tests nutritional deficiencies can be detected, as can endocrine abnormalities and other chronic illnesses.

When a girl has reached sixteen and menarche has still not occurred, this is called "primary amenorrhea." Primary amenorrhea may result from a number of causes. The hypothalamus or pituitary glands may not be functioning normally, in which case the hormones responsible for stimulating the ovaries to influence the lining of the uterus to be shed are not produced. Abnormalities of other glands can affect the ovaries indirectly because of their relationship to the pituitary. The thyroid is the one most often involved; the girl with an abnormal thyroid frequently does not menstruate. Increased production of male hormones by the adrenal glands or by ovarian tumors can also prevent menarche. Very rarely, the ovaries, uterus, or vagina may fail to develop. A disorder of chromosomes, the genetic material which determines sex as well as all other traits, may also be responsible. Methods are now available for evaluation of this rare possibility.

It has been our experience that primary amenorrhea is seldom the first indication of a serious disorder. More often the physician has been alerted to the underlying problem by the presence of other symptoms of the disorder which appear prior to adolescence. Moreover, most of the conditions described can be corrected by surgery or appropriate hormone treatment. Even in the very rare situation where ovaries are absent, resulting in sterility, hormones can be administered to produce monthly bleeding and keep the patient from feeling different from her peers.

The more frequent menstrual abnormality is secondary amenorrhea. This term is used to describe the situation in which a girl who has previously menstruated regularly ceases to do so for a period of more than three months. Endocrine imbalance or tumors of the pituitary, hypothalamus, adrenal glands, or ovaries can be responsible for this condition, as well as for primary amenorrhea. In our experience recently, however, the most frequent cause for secondary amenorrhea has been some form of drug abuse. Fully one-third of the girls we have examined who were using heroin have had this problem. Apparently this phenomenon is a well-known part of the drug subculture. We have had many girls come to us for assistance because their periods did not return after they stopped using drugs, rather than for amenorrhea while on drugs, which they accept as normal. This prolonged amenorrhea, even after drugs are stopped, is cause for concern, because no one knows yet what the long-range effect of drug use on ovulation will be. LSD and amphetamines as well as heroin are known to cause secondary amenorrhea. Some tranquilizers, even when used as prescribed rather than abused, have also caused this problem, so that a complete history of medication use is taken when a patient comes to the doctor.

Most sexually active teen-agers who stop menstruating automatically assume that they are pregnant. Tragedy may result when a girl faced with this problem is frightened into seeking the help of a criminal abortionist rather than a physician. It is important that girls realize that there are many other reasons for secondary amenorrhea, most of which are curable.

If too vigorous a "scraping" or curettage of the uterine cavity has been performed to diagnose a bleeding disorder, amenorrhea may result. This can also result from a criminal abortion.

The Stein-Leventhal syndrome, characterized by hirsutism, obesity, and polycystic ovaries, can cause amenorrhea. For some unknown reason an operation in which a wedge is removed from the ovary will often result in menstruation and fertility. Once the diagnosis of Stein-Leventhal syndrome has been made, it is best to wait for the time that conception is desired to perform this operation.

Women in concentration camps frequently stopped menstruating. Whether it was the psychological trauma alone that was responsible, or whether the poor nutrition of the prisoners also contributed is difficult to determine. We do know that planned dieting can also cause secondary amenorrhea.

Dysmenorrhea

Menstrual cramps are not emotional in origin. They do not result from poor preparation for womanhood. Physiologic studies have demonstrated strong and irregular contractions of the muscles of the uterus at the time when such cramps are experienced. Since these muscular contractions have been found both in girls who did and girls who didn't suffer from cramps, the difference probably lies in the threshold for perceiving pain. Further studies indicate that the hormone progesterone is responsible for the contractions. Progesterone is produced by the corpus luteum which is formed each time an egg is released by the ovary. On the basis of these findings, it is not difficult to understand the reason that the first few menstrual periods in the adolescent are usually pain-free. No egg is produced in these early periods. As a result, there is no corpus luteum and, hence, no progesterone. Many young girls falsely interpret the early absence of cramps as a sign that they will continue to enjoy painless periods and are frequently dismayed to discover that such is not the case.

In addition to physiological factors that cause discomfort to a greater or lesser extent in all teen-agers, there are a few specific structural abnormalities that may also cause menstrual cramps. Severe cramps associated with scanty menstrual flow and present from the time of the first period may be the result of an incomplete opening of the cervix. Monthly cramps in the absence of any external signs of bleeding in a young adolescent may result from an imperforate hymen which blocks the outpouring of menstrual bleeding, a condition called hematocolpos, which requires surgical correction. Infection of the fallopian tubes can also cause menstrual cramps. Relief will follow adequate treatment for the infection. In women over twenty, but rarely in adolescents, so-called fibroids (non-cancerous tumors of uterine muscle) or endometriosis (implants of the tissue which ordinarily lines the uterine cavity in places other than the uterine cavity) can be responsible for cramps at the time of menstruation.

Once these specific disorders have been ruled out, a diagnosis of physiologic dysmenorrhea is made. Fine, now what do you do about it? Therapy for menstrual cramps can be divided into two categories: medical and do-it-yourself. Both are important and should be part of a comprehensive program. Under the heading of medical come various medications that can be prescribed by the physician. Most doctors will start with the simplest and least toxic medications available. Analgesics such as aspirin and darvon may do the trick. If such is not the case, an anti-spasmodic containing atropine frequently diminishes uterine contractions to a point at which they are no longer perceived as painful. For reasons that are not entirely clear, low doses of amphetamines taken on the first day of the period have been shown to eliminate menstrual cramps. When all medications and other forms of therapy fail and the patient is diagnosed as having severe dysmenorrhea, oral contraceptives may be prescribed. The rationale for such therapy is that by eliminating ovulation, progesterone production will be prevented, and this will usually stop the uterine contractions responsible for the cramps. After three months contraceptive medication is stopped and the patient is re-evaluated.

DO-IT-YOURSELF APPROACH TO PREVENTING MENSTRUAL CRAMPS

Retention of water in the wall of the uterus is thought to contribute to menstrual cramps. Because it has been shown that excess water is retained in the tissues of the pelvic organs in the week prior to the start of a period, the first phase of self-treatment consists of preventing water accumulation. The simplest way to do this is to limit salt intake during this week. Pizza, hot dogs, potato chips, and other salty foods should also be avoided.

While all the medications described above, with the exception of the oral contraceptives, are used to suppress the symptom of pain, none will actually prevent cramps. According to L. J. Golub, M.D., prevention can be accomplished in more than half of dysmenorrhea sufferers by a simple routine of exercise. The following exercises should be started on the day after all menstrual bleeding has stopped. Most girls will note the beneficial effect by the third period.

1. Stand erect with feet 1½ feet apart. Arms are raised sideward at shoulder height.
2. Try to touch your left heel with the fingers of the right hand. This is best done by bending forward at the waist and twisting to the left without bending your knees.
3. Return to erect position. Repeat by trying to touch the right heel with the left hand.
4. Repeat four times in each direction at first, and gradually increase to a total of ten times in each direction.
5. Do entire set of exercises three times a day.

Whatever you do, don't be discouraged. There is something that can be done for every girl with menstrual cramps. It's just a matter of having patience, trying different combinations, and being willing to do some of it yourself.

Abdominal Pain

An old-time general practitioner (who also happens to be my father—I.L.) used to say that pain in a girl's abdomen was the easiest ailment to diagnose. It is either due to the fact that she is having her menstrual period, that she is between periods, or she's not going to have a period again for nine months. Although obviously said with tongue-in-cheek, the statement has merit. We have already discussed the first and third of these, namely dysmenorrhea and pregnancy. Abdominal pain midway between periods is extremely common and deserves some attention. The occurrence of pain at this time is sometimes referred to as *Mittelschmerz*, a German word that literally translates as "pain in the middle."

Mittelschmerz is characterized by a pain on one side of the lower part of the abdomen that lasts for no more than a day and is not accompanied by fever, nausea, loss of appetite, constipation, or diarrhea. In one who is keeping a temperature chart it corresponds to the dip, followed by a rise in temperature at mid-cycle. The normal milky, odorless physiologic vaginal discharge will tend to increase in amount at this time. As indicated in the section on vaginal discharge, a discharge that is yellow and foul-smelling and is associated with lower abdominal pain and fever is probably due to an infection in the ovarian tubes (most often caused by gonorrhea) and is not *Mittelschmerz*.

Mittelschmerz is caused by the release of an egg from the ovary. The resultant tear in the capsule of the ovary is associated with a small amount of bleeding within the peritoneal cavity and causes pain. Depending on one's threshold for pain, she may or may not be aware of it. Those who experience it regularly usually feel it alternate from the right to the left side from month to month. This is because the ovaries alternate in releasing an egg each month.

When this type of pain lasts more than a day, an ovarian cyst may be suspected. This condition can be detected by a rectal or vaginal examination. As most cysts tend to disappear of their own accord within two months, most doctors will not consider surgery until after that. Probably all girls get a cyst at some point in their menstrual careers, but ovaries containing many cysts are abnormal and may result in problems of infertility.

If lower abdominal pain on one side is accompanied by fever, nausea, or vomiting, it may be the result of appendicitis, a twisted ovarian cyst, or an ectopic (tubal) pregnancy. If such symptoms occur, a doctor should be consulted at once, for these conditions require immediate surgery.

Pain in the lower abdomen associated with diarrhea can occur because of a gastrointestinal infection or ulcerative colitis (page 92). Lower abdominal pain associated with painful urination may indicate cystitis or a bladder infection.

Although rare, it is important to mention that tumors of the abdomen can be another cause of pain. In adolescent girls the most common tumor in this area would be one arising from the ovary. Ovarian tumors are usually of the benign (non-malignant) variety. They are often accompanied by other symptoms such as increasing abdominal size, menstrual irregularities, and frequency of urination. When a tumor is suspected, surgery is performed both for diagnosis and treatment.

Vaginal Discharge

Fear that vaginal discharge may mean venereal disease keeps most teen-agers from consulting a parent or doctor until they can no longer bear the itching or painful urination that may result from untreated vaginitis.

There are many non-venereal conditions that cause discharge. The most frequent cause in the adolescent age group is not even an infectious one. It is the normal secretion of the glands that line the wall of the vagina. These glands are under the influence of the ovaries, and therefore become active during puberty.

Their secretions are clear white and may leave an odorless stain on the underpants. Vaginal itching and burning on urination does not result from this type of discharge. One characteristic of this so-called "physiologic" discharge is its tendency to become more profuse midway between periods (the time of ovulation). No treatment is necessary, nor is any effective.

Infectious agents that cause discharge range in size from viruses visible only with an electron microscope to worms easily seen with the naked eye. Treatment must be specific for the responsible organism and is quite different in each case. As a result, the temptation to take the medicine prescribed for someone else's discharge should be avoided, for it is often futile and may even hamper the doctor's ability to make a correct diagnosis subsequently.

It is well known that adolescence is a peak time for vaginal infections. While some (*e.g.,* gonorrhea, herpes) are the direct result of sexual contact in this age group, most others are related to changes that take place in the vagina at puberty. Certain bacteria, which do not produce infection, take up residence in the vagina at this time because of the high estrogen levels. As a result of their metabolism the environment within the vagina becomes more acid. Some of the infection-producing organisms (such as trichomonas) thrive in this acidic surrounding. Contraceptive pills render the vagina more prone to infections with yeast-like germs as well.

A discharge that is yellow, green, brown, blood-tinged, or thick white is the result of infection unless proven otherwise. The same is true for any discharge that has a foul or a strong, sweet odor or causes itching or burning on urination. A doctor must be consulted in these circumstances, with one exception. That is the situation where a tampon has been forgotten and left in place for a period of days. The very foul-odored discharge will usually disappear promptly when the tampon is removed and a few sitz baths are taken.

The most frequent cause of infectious discharge in our clinic is trichomonas. While looking like a comical, hairy, single-celled animal under the microscope, the infection it produces is far from funny. Intense itching and a brownish, yellowish, or greenish discharge are usually found. Treatment with Flagyl is effective over a ten-day period. Although this infection is not always the result of intercourse, the male can become a carrier of this organism and should also be treated.

A white, sweet-smelling discharge resembling cottage cheese probably means a yeast infection (monilia or candida). Intense vaginal itching and burning with urination usually result if this is not treated promptly. While pregnancy and diabetes used to be the most common predisposing events for monilial infections, birth-control pills are now a frequent cause. Vaginal suppositories containing a specific anti-monilial agent called Nystatin are the most satisfactory treatment.

The discharge produced by the gonococcus (gonorrhea) can be indistinguishable from that caused by trichomonas or the herpes virus. It can be yellow, green, or brown. It is usually foul-smelling and may cause itching and burning with urination. It may be the only symptom of the infection or may be accompanied by abdominal pain or fever or both. In contrast to gonorrhea in the male (page 85), which is usually apparent within three weeks after intercourse, in the female no symptoms may be present until months later. Abdominal cramps and fever persisting after the second day of the menstrual period are suggestive of gonorrhea. The discovery of penicillin has changed the outlook for someone with gonorrhea in that the incidence of sterility following infection is now less than previously. On the other hand, new strains of the gonococcus are now emerging that are resistant to penicillin so that treatment is more complex than a "single shot."

More rarely a so-called non-specific vaginitis may be responsible for a white or yellow discharge. In this case a variety of bacteria are found on culture. Treatment consists of suppositories or creams containing sulfur or furacin.

Although pinworms are a frequent cause of vaginal discharge in young girls, they are rarely found in adolescent females. When they are present, itching around the vagina and anus is a prominent symptom. Usually one dose of Povan taken by mouth is sufficient to eradicate the infection in one or two weeks.

Vaginal discharge may be an incidental finding in some diseases which affect the entire body. In scarlet fever it is not unusual to culture the streptococcus from a vaginal discharge. In chickenpox and some other virus infections vaginitis may be the most bothersome symptom.

CHAPTER FIVE

The Anatomy of a Male

BASIC MALE ANATOMY

In contrast to those of the female, the sexual parts of the male are for the most part on the outside of the body and clearly visible. This visibility, unfortunately, instead of resulting in an easier understanding of their function and anatomy results all too often in embarrassment and misconceptions.

Therefore we emphasize once again that the size of the organ has nothing to do with the ability to reproduce or the capacity to experience or to give sexual fulfillment.

The Testes or Testicles

We shall start with the testicles because their dual functions, the production of the male hormone and the production of sperm, though separate, are crucial to the male role. The testicles are two ping-pong-ball-sized structures that lie in a bag—the scrotum—at the base of the penis. The left testicle in persons whose hearts are on the left side hangs lower. It sometimes happens that the testicles may be caught in their normal descent either in the abdomen or in the canal along the junction of the thigh and the abdomen, the inguinal area, so that there may be one or no testicles visible. (See the section on undescended testicles.)

Above the testicles, not visible but easily felt, is a smaller mass that caps the testicle, the epididymis. The epididymis is a series of convoluted tubes through which pass the sperm produced in the testes proper on their way to a longer tube called the vas deferens.

The vas deferens, some two feet in length, winds its way from the testicle along the inguinal region and dips down into the abdomen, where it enters a structure called the ejaculatory duct. Also present in this area are two small saclike structures, the seminal vesicles; a larger gland, the prostate; and a smaller pair of glands called Cowper's gland. Secretions from these glands plus the sperm form an emission called semen.

The Urethra

We are now ready to trace the semen's ultimate course through a tube, the urethra, along the body of the penis to its opening, the meatus, through which at other times urine is emitted. The urethra, in addition to being the final pathway for the semen, is connected to the urinary bladder. During erection and ejaculation its opening into the bladder is blocked by a tiny muscle.

The Penis

The outside of the penis consists of a shaft and a head or glans separated from the shaft by a groove and covered in the uncircumcised male by skin called the prepuce or foreskin.

The shaft of the penis is made up of three spongy cylinders richly supplied with blood vessels. There are two corpora cavernosa and a single central cylinder, the corpus spongiosum, through whose course runs the urethra.

FUNCTIONS

In tracing the functions of the various parts of the male anatomy, it is best to begin with the penis and follow the events that start with excitation, then erection, and end, in the usual course of events in the mature male, in ejaculation. This straightforward happening has produced on the one hand some of the supremest pleasure man is capable of experiencing and on the other hand some of his profoundest miseries.

The head of the penis, the glans, is full of very sensitive nerve endings, receptive to both mechanical stimulation and sensual stimulation. This stimulation results in nerve impulses sent to the walls of the blood vessels in the three spongy cylinders, the two corpora cavernosa and the single corpus spongiosum. The blood vessels in response to the nerve messages dilate and grow wider with the engorged blood. This produces the erection.

This state is referred to as tumescence or inflation and gives a great deal of pleasure mingled with expectancy, a prologue to the sense of ultimate pleasurable release resulting in detumescence or deflation.

The erection is pre-ejaculatory, and ordinarily but, alas, not inevitably is followed by ejaculation. Prolonged erection with its blood-vessel engorgement can produce pain in the penis and the testicles.

Ejaculation takes place as the result of the coordinate contraction of groups of muscles that lie along the course of the urethra and vesicles containing the semen, and results in the expulsion of this fluid under considerable pressure. The penis then rather alarmingly deflates as detumescence occurs.

Care of the Male Organs

The Penis—The circumcised penis requires no special care other than the cleanliness one would ordinarily give other parts of the body. The uncircumcised person (circumcisions are not ordinarily necessary) should be careful to pull back the foreskin daily, first to keep it retractile and second to keep the penis itself clean, particularly the groove between the shaft and the tip where foul-smelling debris called smegma collects.

The Testicles—The sperm-producing capabilities of

the testicles are affected by temperature. Theoretically, at least, constricting underwear or support may raise the temperature and interfere with the production of sperm. The corollary is, of course, untrue, and the reader is strongly advised not to depend on tight underwear as a form of birth control.

Masturbation

I suspect that the old hang-ups about masturbation are somewhat outdated; nevertheless, for those who have not read *Portnoy's Complaint* it may be wise to dispel some of the myths about it.

Masturbation used to be referred to as self-abuse, the implication being that it is somehow harmful. The history of this point of view is of some interest. Doctors at the turn of the century noted that insane persons engaged in frequent, and at times public, masturbation. Confusing cause and effect, they wrongly concluded that masturbation caused mental illness. Male and female masturbation is practically universal. It is without consequence and represents a normal developmental phenomenon or the unavailability of an acceptable sexual partner. In and of itself it is not harmful.

Occasionally a fair amount of masturbation may result in the appearance of small amounts of blood, microscopic or barely visible, in the urine. I mention this because ignorance of this fact may result in misdiagnosis and unnecessary tests.

Erections

There are causes of erection other than sexual stimulation. Erections are noted from birth to senescence, when awake and during sleep. They are known to occur during REM or dreaming-state sleep. An irritating foreskin may be a cause of erections. Straining during a bowel movement or lifting heavy objects may result in partial erection. Erection means simply that the spongy tissue in the penis is inflated with blood, and this obviously may occur from a variety of causes.

Wet Dreams

They are not unusual; indeed it is a common occurrence for a man, particularly a young one, to awake in the morning and find himself covered with semen. Since in an ordinary ejaculation this may be as much as a quarter-teaspoonful, it is quite apparent. Needless to say, the presence or absence of emissions during sleep bears no relationship to either the mental health or the sexual potency of anyone.

On Circumcision

Many American children are circumcised at birth; however, with increasing medical resistance to this operation because it is not usually necessary, uncircumcised males are becoming much more common.

It is not unusual to receive a request from an adolescent boy for a circumcision. There are many reasons for such a request, some of them medically valid, others not.

One medically valid reason for a circumcision is the occurrence of what is called a paraphimosis. This occurs when the incompletely retracted foreskin becomes tightly wrapped around the shaft of the penis with resultant swelling and pain. The swelling is not easy to reduce and requires medical assistance. Once this has occurred, a circumcision is probably best.

A second more common but preventable problem is that of phimosis, not to be confused with the previously mentioned paraphimosis. In this situation the foreskin cannot be retracted at all, but becomes fixed at the head, or glans, of the penis. There may or may not be difficulty in urination. If true phimosis exists, that is if the foreskin cannot be pulled back, circumcision is usually recommended.

Most circumcisions can be avoided if proper care is taken at the time of a bath or shower to pull the foreskin gently back to clean the shaft of the penis carefully. Occasionally, as we have seen, a whitish, foul-smelling material with the unpleasant name of smegma is found. This can be easily removed with a washcloth or cotton and is not a reason for performing a circumcision.

PAIN IN THE GROIN

Overlooking pain in the groin or the surrounding areas may have serious consequences. Here again our point is not to make diagnosticians out of you, but to point out logically and factually why certain symptoms demand attention.

Twisting or Torsion of the Testicles

Occasionally, more commonly if the testicle is undescended, the cordlike structure containing the blood-vessel supply to the testicle will become twisted. The result is immediate pain in the testicle, swelling, and, if not corrected surgically within a short time, gangrene. Therefore, to prevent destruction of the testicle, pain in this region should be reported immediately to a physician.

More common, fortunately, is a condition of twisting or torsion of a small structure on top of the testicle, the appendix testicle, a situation, though painful, not nearly so serious as torsion of the testicle proper.

Hernias

A hernia, a bulge of the abdominal contents through a weak place in the abdominal wall, becomes painful only if caught and the blood supply reduced. Such a condition requires immediate medical attention to avoid gangrene. Whether painful or not, a hernia should be treated surgically.

Swollen Glands in the Groin

There are glands, or more properly, lymph nodes that serve as drainage sites for infection for the structures in the leg or the groin region. Consequently any infection in these areas can result in a painful inflammation of the node in the groin. The swelling may vary from the size of a corn kernel to that of a plum. Antibiotics are usually helpful.

UNDESCENDED TESTES

As you will recall, the testicles (testes) migrate from the abdomen to the scrotum and are normally situated at birth in 95 percent of boys. By the time of adolescence one boy in 500 may, if it has not been previously corrected (see below), have one or both of his testicles in an abnormal position outside of the scrotum. Some testes descend naturally between birth and adolescence.

At this point it may be wise to issue a word of warning. Before one can say that the testes are truly in an abnormal position, that is, have failed to make their normal descent, a careful examination, perhaps repeated examinations, may be necessary. The reason for this is that there are testicles that are migratory: they can move up and down from the scrotum to the groin or inguinal region, but are in reality normally placed.

The truly abnormally placed, or undescended, testicle is a cause for concern for several reasons: if allowed to remain in its abnormal position, it will not effectively produce sperm; 2) it is more susceptible to twisting or torsion; 3) some findings indicate that it may be at some greater risk of forming a dangerous tumor. Cancer appears to be more likely to develop in the undescended testicles.

If it is suspected that one or both testicles are not in their normal position, it is not cause for shame nor a reflection on one's manhood, but a reason for investigation of a readily correctable condition.

At present there are different opinions as to when and how undescended testes should be corrected.

If the undescended testicle is in the abdomen or outside of its normal anatomical pathway or if it is associated with a hernia, almost all authorities feel that surgery usually is indicated before five years of age.

When, however, there is merely failure of descent, there are various approaches. One is to give hormones, usually at about five to six years of age, over a four-week period, and if this fails, to operate. Another approach is to operate at age five or six without prior hormone treatment on the theory that hormones are rarely if ever effective. The operation is very safe, regularly successful, and requires about one week in the hospital. A third approach is to wait for puberty, that is, until hair appears around the genitals, before operating in the expectation that many if not all previously undescended testicles will descend at that time.

CHAPTER SIX

The Consequences

AN OUNCE OF PREVENTION . . .

The decision whether or not to have intercourse before marriage is an individual one. Into it goes a background of parental values and religious training onto which is superimposed the example of peers, the desire to prove maturity, love, the desire to become pregnant, impulses and/or impairment in rational thinking such as that caused by alcohol or drugs. Most of the time the decision is spontaneous, and those involved rarely can recall what, if any, thought processes went into it. For adults to say that premarital intercourse is wrong and leave it at that is to evade their responsibility. To condemn attempts by others to educate about contraceptive methods on the grounds that this will invite promiscuity is naïve. It has never been shown that learning about contraceptives ever caused anyone to have intercourse for the first time. Conversely, sexual activity was a problem, albeit not as well publicized, before contraceptives were available. Unfortunately, lack of contraceptives rarely proves a deterrent to sexual activity.

As physicians we are deeply concerned about the health hazard imposed by pregnancy in the teen-ager. This hazard exists for both the pregnant adolescent and her child. This baby is more likely to be born underweight and undersize and therefore has a poorer chance for survival. The teen-ager is more likely to have a stillbirth than the older mother. Indeed, the pregnant girl under fourteen years of age has double the chance for producing a dead infant than one in the fifteen-to-nineteen age group. A baby born to a mother under fifteen years of age has only one-third the chance of surviving infancy of one born to a woman in her twenties.

The pregnant teen-ager runs a great risk of developing toxemia, a condition that produces high blood pressure, convulsions, and even death. She is four times more likely to develop this complication than the pregnant woman over twenty years of age. Because of fear and feelings of shame, she is also less likely to seek early and adequate prenatal care. As a result she frequently becomes nutritionally deficient and anemic.

In addition to these very concrete dangers of teenage pregnancy are those that are more difficult to measure—particularly the psychological effect of such a pregnancy on the girl, her family, and eventually her child.

Another consideration is the threat to life imposed by attempts at criminal abortion. It is well-known that teen-agers comprise the largest percentage of customers for abortionists. In New York City alone more than twenty young girls die each year as a result of criminal abortion, many more than die from pregnancy alone. Hopefully new abortion laws in many states will result in fewer criminal abortions being performed.

In summary, considerations for birth control for teen-agers are different than for adults. While pregnancy itself poses a negligible threat to an adult, this is not the case with a teen-ager. Accordingly, the danger to teen-agers from contraceptive agents must be weighed against the danger of their becoming pregnant.

METHODS OF CONTRACEPTION
FOR THE MALE

Condom

A rubber sheath placed over the penis prior to the sexual act. It is available from the drugstore without a prescription. Leakage of sperm as a result of the condom's cracking or of its slipping off when the penis is withdrawn from the vagina after intercourse is the major drawback to its use. Moistening with vaseline after the condom is in place may prevent cracking, and holding the rim firmly while the penis is withdrawn should avoid its slipping off.

Coitus Interruptus

The method by which the penis is withdrawn from the vagina just prior to ejaculation to avoid introducing sperm into the vaginal canal. The problem with this is that timing is of utmost importance and one can get "carried away" and forget to withdraw in time. In addition, a few sperm may escape before the perceptible sensation of ejaculation and cause pregnancy.

Vasectomy

A surgical procedure in which the sperm cords are tied. Since this is usually an irreversible procedure, it is normally reserved for older men who have already had all the children they desire.

METHODS OF CONTRACEPTION
FOR THE FEMALE

Rhythm System

This requires complete knowledge of the physiology of the menstrual cycle, which is something all girls should know anyway. In essence this method is based on the fact that you can only become pregnant if you have intercourse within the three days before and after ovulation. A good guide to when ovulation occurs is a basal-body-temperature curve, a record of the temperature of the body in the resting state. This is found by taking rectal temperature every morning before arising and recording it accurately. The day prior to ovulation there is a temporary fall in temperature. The day of ovulation temperature rises. The problem with this method (the only one approved by the Catholic Church) is that anything that causes fever will render a temperature curve worthless. The fact that ovulation time varies from one month to the next makes it necessary to keep a record each month. Most teen-agers are not motivated to take their temperature each morning, and many are fearful that the thermometer may be found by a family member at the bedside where it must remain in order to take accurate basal temperature.

Diaphragm

A thin rubber cup with a flexible rim that is inserted into the vagina so that it covers the opening of the cervix. It must be fitted by a physician and refitted after a pregnancy. One young patient became pregnant after she borrowed a friend's diaphragm, a practice to be condemned for many reasons. A diaphragm is lubricated with jelly that kills sperm on contact. Accordingly, it is a safe method of contraception. Young girls profess not to like the diaphragm, claiming that it is too messy because of the jelly. In addition, its use implies expectation of intercourse, and most teen-ages prefer to think of it as spontaneous and unplanned. If used, it must be kept in place for at least eight hours after intercourse.

Foam

A spermicidal foam is available in drugstores without prescription. It is introduced into the vagina with an applicator within the hour prior to intercourse and is fairly effective as a contraceptive. It is almost foolproof if used in conjunction with a condom. The fact that the foam turns to a liquid at body temperature, makes it unacceptable to many girls. The same criticisms of premeditation apply as with the diaphragm.

Intrauterine Device

A plastic or metal coil or ring that is inserted within the cervix by a doctor in his office, and must also be removed by him. Some pain and bleeding may follow insertion, but this is usually short-lived. It is not known how or why they work, but IUDs are unquestionably effective in preventing conception. They have the advantage of remaining in place at all times, so that planning for intercourse is not necessary. Because it is difficult to insert an IUD in the cervix of a woman who has never been pregnant, and because these women have a high incidence of pain, bleeding, and actual loss of the coil, it is not advisable in this group. Its presence cannot be detected by the sexual partner.

Oral Contraceptives

By referring to all oral contraceptives as The Pill, the mass media have created much confusion and, we dare say, many "misconceptions." Under this heading have been lumped over twenty-five preparations containing different combinations of estrogens and a progestin. It is vital to make these distinctions because the possible side effects and potential toxicity vary with the dosage of the various components, particularly the estrogen. Another effect of this generalization has been that some teen-agers take whichever pills they can obtain from friends over the course of one month. All available preparations have in common the ability to inhibit ovulation at the level of the master gland, the pituitary, to render the uterine lining unreceptive to implantation by an egg if it does get fertilized, and to thicken the mucous of the cervix to form a kind of barrier to the entry of sperm. Oral contraceptives are available at the pharmacy by prescription only, and they require motivation to be taken each day. They have the advantage that their use is unrelated in time and place to the sexual act.

If side effects do occur, they are similar to those of pregnancy (e.g., nausea, breast fullness, a bloated feeling, fluid retention, and increased vaginal discharge) and usually pass after a few months of use of the pills. If they persist, another preparation with a different dose of hormones can usually be found that is better tolerated by the individual. All preparations predispose to yeast and fungal infections of the vagina.

As with most medications, the effect on the still growing and changing adolescent appears to be different from that on the more static adult. We are indebted to Dr. Leon Falik for this description of differences of the effect of oral contraceptives on these two groups:

Within six months after stopping oral medication, eighty to ninety percent of adult women will return to a normal pattern of ovulation. In adolescent females, however, only forty-five to fifty percent will return to normal ovulation in this same period of time. In adults, those who did not ovulate normally within the six-month period will do so after one year. This is in contrast with the teen-age girls, thirty percent of whom require one to one and one-half years before returning to normal.

In order to make some sense out of the twenty-odd preparations of oral contraceptives, they can be divided into two main groups. The first is the *combination pill,* which contains, as the name implies, a combination of estrogen and progestin. The same pill is taken for twenty or twenty-one days, depending on the particular pill, and then stopped. About three days after the last pill, withdrawal bleeding will occur that appears like normal menses and lasts about five days. On the fifth day of menses, pill taking is resumed on a daily basis.

The second type of pill is the *sequential pill,* in which the estrogen and the progestin are contained in separate pills that are taken in sequence over the course of the month. With this method a pill is taken every day of the month. Because the latter system more closely simulates the normal hormone production of the menstrual cycle, it would appear that this would be the preferable kind of preparation. However, the sequential pill has been implicated as being more responsible for clotting as a side effect than the combination pill. It also appears that escape ovulation, with resultant pregnancy, occurs more often with this form of therapy.

All oral contraceptives are potentially dangerous in women or girls with migraine headaches, thrombosed veins, and diabetes, for they may aggravate these conditions. The advisability of using them should always be the physician's decision. Their theoretical risks should always be weighed against the very real risks of pregnancy itself in the adolescent.

Some teen-agers believe that one pill taken around the time of intercourse will prevent pregnancy. This is dangerously incorrect. Pregnancy can be prevented only if ovulation is inhibited, which cannot be accomplished unless a pill is taken every day for three weeks after the end of each menstrual period.

ABORTION

New laws in many states now make abortion available to teen-agers. All require permission by one parent unless the girl is emancipated, which generally means that she is married, lives alone, or is self-supporting. If help is desired in interpreting these laws, the offices of Planned Parenthood (listed in the Appendix) are available for that purpose.

Most pregnant girls are understandably afraid to tell their parents of their predicament. It has been our experience, however, that such fears are usually unwarranted. No parent has not himself made a mistake, and few will insist that their daughter pay for hers by having an unwanted baby, unless they do so on the basis of religious belief.

If an abortion is performed by a licensed doctor in a reputable hospital, it is a safe procedure. Abortion does not interfere with the ability to become pregnant in the future. The technique selected by the doctor for abortion is determined by the stage of the pregnancy, that is, how far along it is. In general, it is easiest to have an abortion in the early stages.

Within the first twelve weeks from the day of the last menstrual period, the procedure of choice is dilatation and curettage, commonly referred to as a D&C or "scraping." For this procedure the patient is first put to sleep, after which the cervix is dilated through the vaginal opening so that there is no incision. The products of conception that line the inner wall of the uterus are scraped away with an instrument called a curette or sucked out with a vacuum catheter. The patient is usually permitted to leave the hospital the following day. If desired, an intrauterine device may be inserted at the time of this procedure to prevent future unwanted pregnancies.

In the period between the twelfth and the sixteenth week after the last menstrual period, a hysterotomy may be performed in an adult woman who also is desirous of being sterilized by having her tubes tied. A hysterotomy is a surgical procedure in which the uterus is incised and the products of conception removed just as in a cesarean section. Since this is a major surgical procedure with definite operative risk and no reputable doctor would agree to sterilize a teen-ager, we can conclude that there is no safe abortion procedure for a teen-ager with a twelve-to-sixteen-week pregnancy.

The safest method for abortion in the period between sixteen and twenty-four weeks after the last menstrual period is the saline infusion, commonly referred to as "salting out." A small area of skin on the abdomen is "put to sleep" with an injection of xylocaine, similar to that used by the dentist. Through this anesthetized spot a needle is introduced into the amniotic sac, the fluid-filled bag that surrounds the fetus. The amniotic fluid is drawn out, after which sterile salt water is injected. This initiates labor, and within twenty-four hours the non-living fetus and the placenta are passed spontaneously through the vagina. As with the D&C, there is no incision, stitches, or scar as a result. The patient is usually permitted to leave the hospital the following day.

Most doctors will not perform an abortion after the twenty-fourth week because of the chance that a live infant may be born. In fact, most state laws forbid abortion beyond the twenty-fourth week. If an unwanted pregnancy has continued to that point, it is preferable to arrange for adoption through an established agency.

VENEREAL DISEASE

In the time it took you to sit down and open to this page (two minutes) another teen-ager in the United States contracted VD. VD is the abbreviation for a group of infections caused by contact between genital organs, the so-called venereal diseases. While the usual cause is heterosexual activity, these diseases can also result from homosexual contact. The legendary toilet seat is not a source of VD because the organisms responsible are quite delicate and die immediately after leaving the warmth and moisture of the human genital tract.

Even with underreporting by the medical profession, VD is now rated as the most frequently occurring contagious disease in this country after the common cold. The U.S. Public Health Service reports that after a five-year decline, syphilis has suddenly increased in incidence, especially in teen-agers. Gonorrhea has experienced a steady increase in incidence over the present decade. The rise in number of cases of VD appears to be occurring in adolescents in other parts of the world as well. In Denmark, which is generally considered to have the most advanced system of health care, the problem is no different.

Many theories have been advanced to explain the rise in VD in teen-agers. Lack of sex education in schools; the "new morality" with the vanishing "double standard"; increased prostitution fostered by the need to maintain an expensive drug habit; lack of funds available to public health services for adequate detection of contacts of those with known VD; and widespread use of oral contraceptives rather than condoms, which give mechanical protection against infection, have all been implicated as possible causes.

One factor that appears to contribute to the time interval between infection and cure, and consequently to the period of contagion, is fear of parental detection. In recognition of this observation many states, including New York most recently, have passed legislation allowing doctors to treat teen-agers with VD without parental permission.

Many adults became blasé about gonorrhea and syphilis after the discovery of penicillin in the 1940s. If they were unfortunate enough to contract VD, they reasoned, a shot of penicillin would do the trick. While this attitude may be justified under certain circumstances, we have learned that this wonder drug is not the entire answer. Indeed, it is now apparent that strains of gonorrhea have developed that are resistant to the action of penicillin. At the present time they are found mainly in Southeast Asia, but with GIs returning from Vietnam, it should not be long before they are commonly seen. In addition, a practice of self-administration of a few tablets of penicillin by those who think they are in the know has resulted in suppression of symptoms and interference with tests for syphilis, while allowing the infection to spread unnoticed.

Most teen-agers are not blasé about VD, but rather, uninformed. The boy with an obvious syphilis chancre who explained that he must have caught his penis in his fly while dressing, another who thought it resulted from a cigarette burn, and third who indignantly denied that he could have VD because he only dated girls from "good" families all illustrate the point. It is hoped that the following review of the venereal diseases will fill in some of the gaps.

GONORRHEA

This very common disease is caused by a microscopic bacterium called *Neisseria gonorrheae*. Diagnosis is made upon finding the pink, bean-shaped culprit in stained specimens in microscopic examinations of pus from the genital tract. There is no blood test or easy screening procedure for detecting gonorrhea.

The male who becomes infected develops symptoms within a week after intercourse. The first symptom is the sensation of burning with urination. A non-venereal urinary-tract infection can also produce this sensation. Since both require prompt medical care, anyone with urinary burning should see a doctor immediately. The next symptom is the appearance of pus draining from the penis. It is because of this that gonorrhea is referred to as "the runs" or "the whites." (It is also called "the clap" and "the strain.") A few

boys develop blood in their urine or have difficulty
passing any urine. Because these symptoms disappear,
even without treatment, within two months of their
onset, many mistakenly believe they are cured. Quite
to the contrary, for if untreated, gonorrhea can cause
a permanent narrowing of the urethra, the tube that
leads from the urinary bladder to an opening on the
penis. It can also travel into the epididymis or sperm
ducts, resulting in a hard swelling in the scrotum and
occasionally even sterility.

In contrast to the dramatic symptoms in the male,
gonorrhea in the female may go entirely unnoticed.
While a discharge from the penis is always abnormal,
a girl may have a pre-existing physiologic discharge
(see page 63) and be completely unaware of a superimposed gonorrheal infection. The two can be distinguished, however, in that the former is clear, white,
and odorless, and causes no itching or pain on urination, whereas the latter is usually green, brown, or
yellow, has an unpleasant odor, and does cause irritation. If unnoticed and untreated in this stage, the infection smolders and the girl can infect many partners
without even knowing it. At some point in time, usually at the time of a menstrual period, the bacterium
may gain entrance to the lining of the uterus. From
there it can extend up to the fallopian tubes, where
it causes pain. The pain is experienced as right-
and/or left-sided lower abdominal discomfort. If
right-sided and accompanied by fever, as it frequently
is, the symptoms may be misinterpreted as appendicitis. If not properly diagnosed and treated at this stage,
the fallopian tubes may become blocked with pus, resulting in sterility. Other complications include pelvic
abscess and abnormal menstrual bleeding. It is important to emphasize that whereas the male with gonorrhea knows it within one week of contracting the infection, the female may be infected for months before
she notices symptoms. Because of this, control of gonorrhea by contact detection is nearly impossible.

In both sexes gonorrhea may cause an infection of

one or more joints, a form of arthritis. An individual under treatment for gonorrhea remains contagious until therapy is completed, and obviously should therefore refrain from having intercourse.

Unless a resistant strain is detected, the drug of choice for gonorrhea is penicillin. It is usually administered in a series of four injections, divided so that two are given upon diagnosis and two a week later. Penicillin can also be given in the form of pills to be taken over a ten-day course. The difficulty with this regimen is that most people tend to stop taking their medication after symptoms disappear, frequently an insufficient period for adequate therapy. Penicillin-resistant strains usually respond to ampicillin. Tetracycline is used for those allergic to penicillin. Once the infection has involved the tubes in the female, more vigorous therapy is required and hospitalization may be necessary to effect it. It is important, too, to remember that gonorrhea is not like mumps—you can get it again if re-exposed!

SYPHILIS

"My wounds stink and are corrupt because of my foolishness. For my loins are filled with a loathsome disease; and there is no soundness in my flesh" (Psalms 38:5,7). This passage is interpreted by some to illustrate that syphilis is a disease as old as man. Others argue that it was a disease of the Western Hemisphere, introduced to Europe by Columbus' sailors. Whatever its history, there is no question that syphilis is very much a disease of the twentieth century. It is acquired almost exclusively by teen-agers and young adults in our society. In 1966 one out of every six cases occurred in the fifteen-to-nineteen age group.

Syphilis is caused by the corkscrew-shaped organism *Treponema pallidum,* which can be seen only with the aid of a microscope with a special condenser. The *Treponema* is quite frail, so delicate in fact that it can be destroyed upon contact with ordinary soap and water. It cannot thrive outside the human body. For a long time syphilis was difficult to diagnose because of its fragility and the special equipment necessary for viewing it. Fortunately these obstacles have been overcome by the development of simpler tests that detect the antibodies to the *Treponema* in the blood of the infected individual. The blood examination required before marriage in most states is one such test. These laws have been enacted because a mother with syphilis can pass it on to her unborn child, resulting in the child's death or severe deformity. The only other way syphilis is spread from one individual to another is by sexual contact.

The first sign of syphilis is the chancre, a painless, hard sore that appears from ten to ninety days after exposure. The chancre is usually found near the tip of the penis, so it rarely goes unnoticed by the infected male. In the female, however, the chancre commonly occurs on the cervix. Its location and the fact that it is painless make self-detection unlikely in girls. Disappearance of the chancre does not mean cure, for this will occur within three to five weeks even with no treatment, only to reappear in a different form weeks later. The secondary form of syphilis consists of fever, rash, patchy baldness, and/or shiny bumps in the genital area. These symptoms will also disappear without therapy, usually within months to a year later. Syphilis is highly contagious in the first and second stages. The third stage is not seen in teen-agers, for it occurs years after the initial infection. This stage is characterized by progressive deterioration of the nervous and cardiac systems and results in incapacitation and death.

In the first and second stages of syphilis, diagnosis can be made by demonstrating the *Treponema* in scrapings from the chancre or skin lesions. Blood tests assist in diagnosis, especially in the period between the symptomatic stages, when physical examination may be entirely negative. Treatment consists of four injections of penicillin, two given at diagnosis and two a week later. Treatment of tertiary syphilis requires more extensive penicillin therapy. Tetracycline is usually prescribed for those allergic to penicillin.

THESE "LOUSY" KIDS

The recent rise in the incidence of *Phthirus pubis* (pubic or crab lice) in teen-agers suggests that more than flowers are passed around at love-ins. Infestation with pubic lice is another venereal disease, for it usually results from sexual intercourse. Unlike gonorrhea and syphilis, however, it can occasionally be transmitted through intimate contact with the bedclothes of an infested person.

The crab louse attaches to a pubic hair and pierces the surrounding skin. It may also settle down in other hairy regions if mechanically transported there. The eggs, or nits, are also firmly attached to the hair near the skin. They are so small as to escape detection with the naked eye. Their presence is suspected if a person has an intense itch in the pubic area, and diagnosis is confirmed by microscopic examination. Although the louse is not itself a carrier of disease, the irritated area produced by scratching can become secondarily infected. The louse bite frequently produces small hemorrhages in the skin, called "sky-blue spots."

A lotion, cream, or shampoo containing gamma benzene hexachloride (such as Kwell or Topocide) is a simple and effective treatment. Because of the frequent coexistence of other, more serious venereal diseases, a complete physical examination is indicated in anyone infested with "crabs."

CHAPTER SEVEN

The Ills Their Flesh
Is Heir To

The purpose of this section is not so much to present the information necessary to make a differential diagnosis, nor to practice do-it-yourself medicine, but rather to encourage periodic visits to a physician. Granted that adolescents resist going to a physician. Granted too that exhortation to do so would probably be unavailing. We hope, nevertheless, that a straight presentation of some of the illnesses more likely to occur in adolescence than at any other time will result in more rather than fewer visits to a doctor as a result of the instinct for self-preservation if not out of intellectual curiosity. Adolescence is a time of stress, both physiological and psychological. It is not to be inferred, however, that the illnesses discussed below are the direct result of that stress, but merely that stress plays some role in their onset. As a matter of fact, the specific causes of all of these illnesses are unknown.

DIABETES MELLITUS OR
"SUGAR DIABETES"

A typical story. John, aged fifteen, has been seemingly well. He notices, however, that he has to urinate more frequently than previously. As a matter of fact, he has to get up during the night to do so.

He soon finds that he is drinking more water, because "I am thirsty all the time." The frequent urination is not painful, just inconvenient. The thirst is easily relieved, so he doesn't worry about it. His appetite is good, but nevertheless he is losing weight. If he has enough sense at this point to visit the doctor, a simple urinalysis and some confirmatory blood tests for determining the amount of sugar in the blood will make the problem apparent. Should he, however, ignore these symptoms, the process goes on to graver and sometimes fatal consequences. As a result of having to urinate all the time to get rid of the excess sugar, John gets dehydrated, dried out. In addition, since his body cannot use the sugar, he starts metabolizing fat. The dehydration and the reliance on fat as a source of energy result in a state of diabetic acidosis. Its symptoms are drowsiness, nausea, and vomiting. At this point John feels pretty damn sick. But even now the medical management is not difficult. If neglected at this relatively late stage, however, coma is sure to follow. There is no doubt about seeing a doctor then.

At this point John's life is in jeopardy. But thanks to insulin and our knowledge of the proper use of fluids, practically all diabetics can be saved.

It has been our experience that teen-agers are often resistant to treatment for diabetes. Although some of this is psychological—the adolescent's fear of being different, his resistance to adult direction, his reawakened sense of omnipotence—the task may be made unnecessarily difficult because of misinformation.

A diabetic *can* lead an absolutely normal life. Only his doctor need know. In the first place, no special diet is required. Most physicians now feel that the so-called free diet is best. A free diet does not imply a capricious diet. It is free but sensible. Its guidelines are precisely those that one would hope a teen-ager without diabetes would follow. There are no restrictions on sweets. Desserts, ice cream, and candy all are okay. This may seem surprising. It is only fairly recently that many doctors have concluded that in the short as well as the long run, persons with diabetes do just as well whether they are on restricted, measured diets or not.

Furthermore, it is now felt that it is perfectly all

right to spill moderate amounts of sugar in the urine as long as there is no excessive urination, thirst, or weight loss.

The keystone in the management of diabetes is insulin, a hormone secreted by the pancreas that is necessary for the use of sugar for energy by the body cells. The diabetic pancreas secretes either inadequate insulin or none at all. Unfortunately, practically all teen-agers with diabetes must take insulin by injection rather than oral medication. The modern insulins usually require administration once a day—at most twice. The technique is readily mastered, and even variations in dosage can be learned.

What was once an untreatable and often fatal disease has become readily manageable, imposing on its victims practically no encumbrances to a normal life.

ULCERATIVE COLITIS

Although this disease is relatively rare, it is worth talking about, since it is a disease primarily of young adults. The cause is unknown. We understand what it is, but not how it comes about. It is, as its name implies, an inflammation of the colon, that is, the large bowel. In contrast to ordinary inflammations due to viruses, bacteria, parasites, all of which a doctor will consider before he arrives at his diagnosis, ulcerative colitis is a chronic disease of long duration, characterized by periods of exacerbation alternating with periods of remission and freedom from symptoms. It may make its appearance in either one of two ways. It can appear as painless—we emphasize *painless*—rectal bleeding, in contrast to the pain and discomfort associated wth the more common ailments such as hemorrhoids (piles) or fissures. Should one experience painless rectal bleeding, it is reason to seek fairly prompt medical attention.

The physician will immediately want to do a rectal examination. This is done by inserting his finger into the rectum to feel for a growth, usually a polyp, which could cause bleeding. If he finds nothing he will want to do a proctoscopic examination. The proctoscope is a tube with a light that can be inserted into the rectum for direct observation of the intestinal wall, called the mucosa. An experienced observer can diagnose ulcerative colitis merely by observation.

The second way the disease presents itself is by abdominal pain with diarrhea, pus, and sometimes blood. When all efforts have been made to rule out all the usual causes of this fairly common symptom complex (bacteria, amoeba, or indirect evidence of virus infection), one begins to suspect ulcerative colitis. It can be confirmed by proctoscopy.

Treatment is complicated. At one time ulcerative colitis was thought to be primarily an emotional disorder. A characteristic personality has been described. The victims are passive, punctilious, oversensitive, and have an excessive need for love. They have been described as overly dependent on their mothers, who in turn are described as cold, domineering, strict, and primitive. The psychological explanations are more facile and interesting than they are helpful.

No one doubts that the disease can be worsened by emotional upset and that many patients benefit from either counseling or psychotherapy, but the true cause is not yet understood. It requires total, comprehensive treatment, description of which is beyond the scope of this book. We reiterate, however, that this illness, or rather the symptoms by which it presents itself, are reasons for seeking medical care.

REGIONAL ILEITIS

Although this disease is relatively rare, it is one more likely to occur in the second or third decades of life. Remember, however, that former President Eisenhower suffered from it. Its symptoms are not dissimilar to those of ulcerative colitis in that it may present abdominal pain and diarrhea. It is often accompanied by fever, so that acute appendicitis may be suspected. It is a disease of the ileum (the lowest part of the small intestine). Local abscesses can cause scarring, producing a thickened, hardened, inelastic, and narrowed intestine. It is a chronic disease, requiring comprehensive medical care.

ASTHMA

Asthma is a disease that usually starts in childhood, but since it is exacerbated by stress, it is included here. It is basically a spasm of the smaller tubes leading to the bronchioles in the lung. The result of this spasm and the resultant narrowing of the bronchioles is that the passage of air, particularly out of the air sacs in the lung, becomes extremely difficult. The patient experiences a sense of tightness and difficulty in breathing, particularly when exhaling, and an audible whistle or wheeze is often heard. There is usually no fever, and the onset, though occasionally preceded by an intractable cough, is usually sudden.

A physician will ordinarily have no difficulty diagnosing asthma.

Its cause is probably multiple. Undoubtedly, there is individual susceptibility to it, based on heredity, but the precipitating events may be infectious, allergic (due to horse hair, feathers, cosmetic powders, pollen, etc.), psychological, or a combination of any or all of these.

Treatment is dependent in part on the frequency and the severity of the attacks, and to a lesser extent on the persuasion of the physician. The management of the acute attack is fairly standard. Medications that will relax the spasm are issued, such as adrenalin by injection. Ephedrine, a compound related to adrenalin, can be given by mouth. It is often prescribed, either alone or in combination with other medication. A barbiturate in small doses to counteract the excitatory effects of the ephedrine is often employed. Xanthine derivatives related to theophylen, the stimulant in tea, are used. The commonest used is aminophyline, administered orally, rectally, or intravenously. These drugs have to be used with caution and should not be overused. Inhalers containing dilators of the bronchial tree are discouraged because patients can easily become dependent on them.

The long-range management of asthma is concerned with removal of the offending allergens or desensitizing the person to them. Asthma beginning in adolescence is usually associated with inhalants, microscopic particles derived from the outer integument of animals (such as horse hair, dog hair, feathers, wool) common house dust, or pollens derived from plants.

The simplest method of averting attack is to avoid these substances, particularly in the sleeping area. Below is outlined the method used to create an allergically clean bedroom, designed more for the asthmatic than the erotic.

Heating:

One of the reasons that allergic conditions frequently worsen during the winter months is the use of heat. Heating systems, particularly hot-air ones, stir up dust. Steam or hot water is preferable to hot-air systems. A dust filter made of several layers of cheesecloth placed over hot-air outlets is helpful. The filter should be changed frequently. Cracks or holes around pipes or radiators should be covered.

The Room:

After the heating system has been checked, the next step is the preparation of the room. Start from scratch. The room should be emptied completely and thoroughly, then cleaned, with special attention given to scrubbing the woodwork to remove all traces of dust. The floor should be waxed.

The room, if possible, should contain only one bed, preferably an iron bed. If box springs are used, they should be enclosed in a dustproof casing. The mattress should have a dustproof cover. No mattress pad should be used; nor should fuzzy wool blankets or feather- or wool-stuffed comforters. There are many adequate blankets or quilts made out of synthetics, such as dacron, that are excellent.

Plain, non-upholstered chairs made of wood or metal are best. We once saw a patient whose asthma was markedly improved when an overstuffed easy chair was removed from his bedroom.

The room should be cleaned and aired daily, after which it should be kept shut.

Clothing, particularly woolens, should be kept in another room. All animals with fur or feathers should be kept out of the room.

Needless to say, the remainder of the house should be kept as dust-free as possible. In general, it is best to keep the house well humidified. Dryness seems to increase the likelihood of infections, which may trigger off allergies, and in addition moisture tends to keep dust down.

Should this method not be effective, desensitization—a series of shots containing increasing amounts of the previously tested-for allergens—may have to be employed. This is a long process, and shots must be continued for a matter of years. The results are usually good.

Occasionally, cortisones have to be used during an acute attack or when asthma is unremitting or intractable. More than likely there will be relief from the use of these preparations. The problem is that the patient may become psychologically dependent on them and they may be difficult to discontinue. There are so many side effects to the cortisone drugs—the steroids, as they are known medically—that if their use cannot be avoided the patient should be under careful medical supervision.

Psychological factors undoubtedly play a part in

precipitating an asthma attack, but it is unlikely that they are the basic cause. Counseling or psychotherapy, however, may be helpful.

SEIZURES, CONVULSIONS, EPILEPSY

The social stigma associated with a convulsion, probably related to its medieval association with evil spirits, has been the cause of much suffering and a good deal of medical neglect.

We have grouped seizures, convulsions, and epilepsy together, for the terms are often used interchangeably, although strictly speaking they are not one and the same thing.

For our purposes a convulsion and a seizure are the same. By definition they are the sudden appearance of some major or fleetingly minor bodily movement associated with some alteration of the state of the consciousness, which may vary from a momentary lapse to complete unconsciousness. A seizure may have a wide variety of causes. It may result from pressure on the brain—a brain tumor or a collection of blood—or an inflammation of the brain such as encephalitis or meningitis. Low blood sugar or low calcium, rarely low magnesium or low sodium, may also cause convulsions, but it is important to point out that this is never merely a dietary deficiency but an indication of some underlying disorder.

If after investigation no particular cause is determined, the only positive finding being an abnormal brain-wave test or EEG (electroencephalogram), we sometimes call the condition epilepsy. It appears, however, that no amount of explaining will remove the horrible connotation of this word from the lay mind. We therefore yield to popular feeling and use the term convulsive disorder.

A major convulsion, known best by the French term *grand mal* ("large sickness") is usually marked by uncontrollable, alternating contractile tightening

and loosening movements of the entire body with falling and loss of consciousness, foaming at the mouth,
and perhaps biting of the tongue and involuntary passage of urine and/or stool. It may be preceded by an
"aura," such as a scene passing through the mind, a
smell, a hallucination of some sort. The entire process
is a reflection of an alteration in the electric rhythm
of the brain waves, much the same as the flickering of
a light bulb when the current has been interrupted.
Rarer during adolescence—as a matter of fact, it usually disappears during this period—is *petit mal* ("little" or "minor sickness"). In this type of seizure are
what appear to be staring spells. The affected person
stares momentarily ahead, may stop talking in the
middle of a sentence, and then, after a moment, resume conversation. He has no memory of the event
and cannot be distracted during this brief episode. *Petit mal* can be easily diagnosed with an EEG.

Treatment of convulsive disorders is by anti-convulsant medication. Well over 90 percent of patients
can be controlled with phenobarbital, which has virtu-
ally no toxic effects if taken as prescribed, and/or Dilantin, which is a relatively safe drug with very few
side effects.

Despite the stigma and the general sense of unpleasant awe associated with convulsive disorders, it
does remain a fact that the overwhelming number of
people so afflicted can be successfully treated and can
lead relatively normal lives. There are some restrictions as to occupation—no service in the army, no
working near open machinery or high places—in addition to some restrictions in obtaining a driver's li-
cense. When there has been freedom from seizure for
a number of years, driving is usually permitted.

HEADACHES

One out of two adolescents suffers at one time or
another from chronic recurrent headaches. These are,

of course, to be distinguished from the single episode of headaches, the kind of headache that may accompany any type of infection and whose course roughly parallels that of the infection, and the occasional solitary headache that we all get from time to time.

The chronic headache that we refer to is the type that comes, lasts for minutes or hours—on rare occasions days or months—either being there constantly or recurring over varying periods of time.

There are many causes of chronic headaches, and anyone suffering from them should see a doctor. The problem is not always simple.

Brain Tumors

Let us start with a life-threatening but fortunately rare cause of headache. The headache caused by a brain tumor may have any location, may be relentless or remitting, and may be associated with memory lapses, awkwardness, clumsiness, uncontrollable movements, or vomiting. Immediate medical attention is necessary.

Migraine

Migraine is far more common than most people, including physicians, are aware. The name is derived from the Latin *hemicrania,* or half-head, vulgarized to migraine. The reason for this name is that classical typical migraine involves one side or half of the head.

The headache of migraine is what is called a vascular headache, that is, having to do with a blood vessel. It begins with the abnormal contraction of a blood vessel—this is called vasospasm—followed by a period of abnormal widening of the blood vessel—called vasodilation.

The brain substance itself is insensitive to pain, but spasms of the blood vessels cause pain by their effect on the nerve endings in the covering of the brain, called the meninges. Migraine occurs in several forms:

CLASSIC MIGRAINE

This is the commonest type and often runs in the family. The headache may be prefaced by some difficulty in vision—a blind spot, a colored ring around a light, or, rarely, the appearance of normal objects as very small. This last phenomenon, where objects look as though they were seen through the wrong end of the telescope, is usually misdiagnosed as some form of hysteria. It is of some interest to note that Lewis Carroll, the author of *Alice in Wonderland,* was himself known to have severe migraine.

These phenomena are usually, but not always, followed by a headache. They represent that stage when the blood vessels going to the brain are abnormally narrowed or in vasospasm. The headache that follows is usually one-sided and severe. During the attack the sufferer will probably want to avoid light and may vomit. The headache, which may last for minutes or hours unless checked by medication, is usually followed by drowsiness.

COMMON MIGRAINE

In common migraine, so-called, the early symptoms are quite vague, a sick feeling or a premonition of a headache. The headache may be one-sided and last for several hours. It is often accompanied by a runny or stuffy nose and may sometimes be confused with a sinus infection. (See below.)

CLUSTER MIGRAINE

Cluster migraine consists of moderate attacks occurring in groups over one-half- to one-and-one-half-hour periods. This is rather unusual in adolescents.

HEMIPLEGIC MIGRAINE

Hemiplegia is Latin for paralysis of one side. As the name implies, hemiplegic migraine is a severe headache followed by transient paralysis of one side of the body, including the lower face, arm, and leg. This can scare the heck out of anybody, including your physician. Fortunately, the paralysis is the result of changes in the caliber of the blood vessel, and will start to clear when the blood vessel returns to normal. This will happen in a matter of hours.

OPHTHALMOPLEGIC MIGRAINE

In this form of migraine the headache is followed by paralysis of the temporarily weakened muscles that move the eyeball around. The eye is abnormally pulled to the stronger muscle side, up or down, in or out, depending on which muscles are affected.

BASILAR ARTERY MIGRAINE

Recently a type of migraine has been discovered peculiar to young girls. The discovery is so recent and the type of migraine so rare that even an experienced physician may have difficulty in recognizing it. Maybe you can help your physician out, but remember to be gentle about it. He is subject to headaches, too, you know.

The blood vessels involved are at the base of the brain, and the symptoms depend on what part of the brain they supply. This type of headache frequently occurs around the time of menstruation. The first thing usually noticed are some blind spots in the field of vision. These are known medically as scotomata. These may be followed shortly after by a feeling of dizziness in which objects in the room seem to be going around the person. There then may occur some difficulty in pronouncing words. Speech becomes slurred. The patient may lose her balance or stagger drunkenly. Occasionally there is a tingling sensation with or without ringing in the ears. These symptoms may last for almost an hour; then they are followed by a severe headache at the base of the skull.

There are very few illnesses that include all of these symptoms; so this kind of headache, if one is aware of it, is not too difficult to diagnose, and can be controlled.

There is a wide variety of drugs that are helpful in migraine. Because one naturally likes to use the simplest drugs with the least side effects, aspirin is first employed at the onset of the attack. If this is not successful, a barbiturate, short-acting so that it gives less of a hangover, is used with the aspirin.

If this is not helpful, a drug called ergotamine, which causes constriction of blood vessels, is used early in the attack in combination with caffeine.

If vomiting occurs, there are anti-emetics, drugs that prevent or control vomiting and can be taken rectally, that are helpful.

If the attacks are frequent and severe, barbiturates such as phenobarbital can be used on a daily basis to prevent them. This treatment is also effective. A relatively new drug called methysergide, also used to prevent attacks, has many side effects and should be used with great caution.

An anti-convulsant called Dilantin has been rarely but at times strikingly helpful in migraine, particularly when there is a family history of convulsions tied in with the migraine. This does not mean that a person with migraine has epilepsy or is even susceptible.

Tension Headaches

A more frequently appearing headache is the so-called tension or nervous headache. The pain is a reflection of increased muscle tension, usually in the muscles in the neck attached to the base of the skull and occasionally in the muscles of the brow and top of head. Tension headache is basically psychological in cause, in contrast to migraine, which is probably either hereditary or constitutional. These headaches may consist of constant pain in the base of the skull, the occiput, or the feeling that one's head is in a vise or that one is wearing a tight cap. The headache can last hours to weeks or months.

Aspirin and mild sedatives are helpful. Momentary freezing of the muscles by a spray or injections of local anesthetic to break up trigger areas of pain have been helpful to some.

Psychotherapy can be extremely helpful in both migraine and tension headaches. By psychotherapy we do not necessarily mean deep psychoanalysis, but occasional guidance in rearranging the facts of one's life. The victims of both types of headaches are, in general, worrisome and conscientious. Often they take on too many extracurricular activities, so that they feel tense and driven. Merely cutting down on some of these activities and having some regard for one's own welfare can often cause surprising results.

Sinus Headaches

A sinus headache is usually a dull, constant ache, usually not severe, over the area of the frontal sinuses, that is, just above the eyes. It will be accompanied by other signs of sinus infection such as nasal congestion. On rare occasions, if the sinuses behind the nose, the spenoid ethmoids, are involved, there may be a headache at the back of the head. Chronic sinusitis is rare in adolescence unless there is accompanying allergic disease or other complicating factors.

The ordinary attack of sinusitis is acute and can be cleared up by antibiotics and medications that shrink mucous membranes.

Headaches from Eye Strain

Eye problems rarely cause real headaches. Annoying pain behind the eyes when reading is usually the only symptom noted. Too often headaches are attributed to poor vision, and sometimes glasses are unnecessarily prescribed for relatively minor visual problems.

In all types of headache good hygiene is important. Sufficient rest, avoidance of drugs and alcoholic beverages, plenty of exercise, and correction of constipation are all helpful. Lastly, let us repeat that anyone with a persistent headache should see a doctor.

HEPATITIS

Yellow eyes and skin, cola-colored urine, and clay-colored bowel movements all combine to paint the picture that is hepatitis. When greeted with this dramatic picture, the victim will not hesitate to seek medical attention. It has been our experience, however, that many teen-agers have hepatitis without ever experiencing these color changes. These are the kids who feel tired all the time and may or may not have a dull pain in the upper part of the right side of their abdomen. Nausea and vomiting are other frequent symptoms.

While it is true that drug-users greatly risk developing hepatitis from unsterilized needles, it does not follow that anyone with hepatitis must be a drug-user. The word hepatitis merely describes an inflammation of the cells of the liver, not a single disease. This inflammation of liver cells results most commonly from infection by a virus found in the blood and transmitted by a needle or transfusion(so-called serum hepatitis); a virus transmitted by saliva or stool ("infectious" hepatitis virus), and another virus that causes infectious mononucleosis or "the kissing disease" (see page 112). Hepatitis may also result from the action of various toxins and drugs such as cleaning fluids, oral contraceptives and antituberculous medications in a sensitive individual. Certain diseases of the arthritis family can also affect the liver and produce symptoms of hepatitis. Moreover, these same symptoms of yellow eyes and skin and stool and urinary changes can result from interference with the flow of bile from the liver. Some anemias or more rarely, a cyst, abscess, gallstone, or tumor can be responsible for this situation.

When a doctor first sees a teen-ager with hepatitis, he will obtain a specimen of blood for chemical tests that indicate the relative extent of damage to the liver cells, and measure the ability of the liver to excrete bile at that point in time. Depending on the results of these tests, he will decide whether or not to hospitalize the patient. It has been our experience that a teen-ager rarely requires hospitalization, so don't be surprised if you are asked to take your yellow-eyed youngster home. The liver-function tests will be repeated at frequent intervals initially, and then less often until they return to normal. Disappearance of the yellow color from skin and eyes and return of stool and urine to their normal color show that the duct system of the liver is no longer obstructed. This is not synonymous with recovery from hepatitis, as destruction of liver cells can go on with no visible consequences. While hepatitis can result in liver failure or hepatic coma and death, most teen-agers recover completely.

The liver is hidden somewhere inside the body (beneath the right side of the rib cage, to be precise), so teen-agers do not as readily identify with it as they do with the organs and structures they can see. We know that they are more concerned with afflictions involving visible parts of their bodies than with potentially more life-threatening diseases of internal organs because the former make them look different from their friends. As a result, once the jaundice has disappeared and they are feeling stronger, they resent limitation of their activity and visits to the doctor's office.

While rest has always been a standing order for patients with hepatitis, recent studies have shown that exercise has no detrimental effect on its outcome. During the contagious phase (approximately one to two months after the onset of symptoms), the patient should be limited to the home and a tutor arranged for, if possible.

Parents frequently ask, understandably, why the patient cannot be hospitalized for the sake of protecting others at home. The fact of the matter is that by the time the patient has developed the symptoms that bring him to the doctor, the family has already been exposed. Don't panic! An injection of gamma globulin will protect those recently exposed. It is only necessary for those people who have eaten with the patient, shared toilet facilities regularly, drunk from his cup, or kissed him on the lips around the time he became symptomatic. The hepatitis virus is probably not passed by conversation. Once family members and fiancés have gotten gamma globulin and the patient has returned home, the following are suggested:

1. Allow activity as desired by the patient.
2. Any food he wants to eat is okay. During the obstructive phase, fatty foods will be shunned. Don't force him to eat—he will when he's ready.
3. Weigh daily and record. Same for temperature. (This will make you feel like you are doing something for him. Actually there is nothing you can do or give that will make any difference.)
4. Use disposable plates, cups, and utensils, and don't forget to discard them after each meal. Have the patient place them in a plastic bag that you can secure with a tie. Disposable toothbrushes are excellent, but expensive. If you prefer not to use them, keep his brush separate with a separate tube of toothpaste in a closed plastic bag. His washcloth and towel should be separated from others. There is no need to wash his things separately, however, for the washing-machine water is hot enough and the virus is probably not hardy enough to survive it.
5. Disposable tissue toilet-seat covers are a good conversation piece, and their use makes most mothers more comfortable about having others share the toilet with the patient. They are usually available in "Bon Voyage" sections of department or drugstores. Toilet-paper strips, though

less glamorous, can serve the same purpose.

6. Things known to damage the liver should be avoided, such as alcohol, various drugs (many tranquilizers, some antidiarrheal pills, oral contraceptives occasionally, antituberculous drugs, and others—best check with the doctor before taking any you are unsure about), and the fumes from cleaning fluids.

"If it can be such a serious disease, why don't you give him a shot or something?" the reasonable parent asks. Unfortunately, as with most other diseases caused by viruses, like the common cold, there is no known drug to combat it. The recent finding of a virus-like particle in the blood of many people with hepatitis makes it possible to hope that a vaccine against the virus may eventually be produced. Some physicians treat hepatitis with cortisone derivatives, but there is little convincing data to indicate that this makes any difference in the course of the disease.

If the liver-function tests have not returned to normal after a few months, most doctors will consider a liver biopsy to obtain first-hand information about the possible long-term effects of the disease. Because of the varying responses to the suggestion of liver biopsy (one boy asked when the liver "autopsy" would take place, and another confused it with a liver "transplant"), let us make clear that it is a simple procedure that can be done in the hospital bed, without anesthesia. A small area of skin (the size of a dime) over the liver is "put to sleep" with an injection of xylocaine, just as is done by the dentist. A larger needle is put through this area into the liver with one quick motion, and a small particle of liver obtained for study. The patient feels only the initial injection of xylocaine and then a sudden pressure sensation when the actual biopsy specimen is obtained. When examined under the microscope, the biopsy specimen can provide information about the extent of damage, the probable course of the disease, and in some instances, the cause of the liver damage.

TONSILLITIS

The tonsil, once regarded as a worthless vestige or even a haven for bacteria, has finally been vindicated. In recent studies children who underwent tonsillectomy following polio vaccination were shown to lack vital antibodies to the polio virus in their nose and throat. Those immunized children who did not have their tonsils removed had adequate protective antibodies in nasopharyngeal secretions. The significance of these observations lies in the fact that in earlier studies Dr. Sabin demonstrated that polio virus may spread directly from the nose and throat to the central nervous system in the absence of adequate local antibody protection.

Even before tonsils were shown to secrete antibodies, doctors had become reluctant to suggest tonsillectomy as a cure for frequent tonsillitis attacks, for they found that once the tonsils were removed, the patient was then bothered by frequent attacks of pharyngitis. Accordingly, it is suggested that tonsillectomy be performed only for the following reasons: (1) frequent middle-ear infection, (2) an abscess of the tonsil, (3) mouth breathing and snoring without other explanation. Whatever its reason, tonsillectomy is never performed during an infection, except in the situation of a tonsillar abscess.

The teen-ager is subject to the same causes of tonsillar infection as the younger child, but in addition, he is more prone to the virus that causes infectious mononucleosis. On the optimistic side, however, during the adolescent years all lymphoid tissue, including the tonsils, undergoes regression.

CHAPTER EIGHT

All That Withers Is Not Soul
—Diseases That Mimic
Emotional Disorders

There are many pitfalls on the climb from childhood to adulthood, not the least of which is the tendency to attribute some hard-to-diagnose physical ailment to the strains and stresses of adolescence.

Thus it is that all that withers is not soul.

Janet, aged sixteen, is feeling tired. It is the end of the semester, and her fatigue is attributed to the strain of preparing for exams. In addition, her appetite is a bit off. This is attributed to worry ("I can't eat when I'm nervous"), and she appears a bit pale ("I guess I don't get enough fresh air"). These common traits of fatigue, poor appetite, and pallor, may be the sign of a number of more or less serious illnesses.

Complaints that are somatic should not be necessarily regarded as psychosomatic. It is difficult to get the adolescent to see a doctor, but perhaps a listing of some of the more common illnesses may be persuasive in encouraging medical investigation of complaints.

ANEMIA

Anemia is a condition that occurs when there is insufficient hemoglobin, the substance in the red blood cell that gives it its color when it carries oxygen to the tissues to sustain life. Hemoglobin itself is composed of two parts: heme, which contains iron, and globin, a complex protein. That's easy so far. The hemoglobin itself becomes incorporated in the red blood cell or red corpuscle, and this unit, the red cell with sufficient hemoglobin, is our oxygen-transport system. When for one reason or another we lack any part of this unit, we are said to be anemic.

It follows that anemia can be due to either a loss of or defective production of hemoglobin or a loss of or defective production of red blood corpuscles. The loss of either substance may be due to bleeding or to destruction in the body.

Given this, it is possible to understand in general that there are various kinds of anemia.

Iron-Deficiency Anemia

Probably the most common deficiency disease in this country at this time is iron-deficiency anemia. A lack of iron in the body results in a hemoglobin deficiency, iron being one of the two constituents of hemoglobin. This deficiency, in turn, is due to either an inadequate intake of iron in the diet or actual blood loss—or, as is the case with many adolescent girls who eat poorly and lose blood by menstruating, it may be due to both.

Bleeding as a cause of hemoglobin loss is obvious; less understood is the role of the diet in anemia.

A diet poor in iron-containing foods results in iron-deficiency anemia. An example of such a diet would be one heavily weighted with: milk products such as ice cream, frosteds, cheeses, and milk; starches such as pizzas, breadstuffs, cakes, pies, and potato chips; and beverages such as sodas or beer—in short, the typical American teen-ager's diet. Foods rich in iron are red meats, eggs, green vegetables, and some fruits, our own favorites being apricots and raisins. How about trying an apricot or raisin pizza the next time?

Most of the varieties of anemia caused by something other than iron deficiency are detectable before adolescence, so we will only touch on them here.

Sickle-Cell Anemia

Sickle-cell anemia is a disease found largely but not exclusively in blacks. It is a result of the inheritance of a defective pattern of hemoglobin synthesis resulting in a red blood cell that, when deprived of oxygen, assumes a sickle shape instead of the normal round shape. This sickle cell in turn sludges and causes poor circulation to the various tissues of the body, resulting sometimes in tissue destruction.

Mediterranean Anemia

Mediterranean anemia, like sickle-cell anemia, is due to an inherited pattern of defective hemoglobin synthesis. It occurs most often but not exclusively in peoples with Mediterranean origins, predominantly Italians. It is recognized usually by malformations of the red cell, which may be seen on a smear of blood on a microscope slide that has been stained.

Leukemia

Leukemia is wild multiplication of the white blood cells. This prevents formation of red cells in adequate numbers, resulting in anemia. Contrary to popular fantasy, the white blood cells do not "eat up" the red cells, but the effect is the same.

G-6-PD Deficiency

G-6-PD is the acronym for an enzyme normally present in red blood cells that prevents their destruction. An individual with G-6-PD deficiency may not know he has it until brought into contact with such otherwise innocuous substances as fava beans or camphor, or more rarely, such medications as sulfa drugs, or even aspirin in large quantities.

All anemias have common symptoms. The lack of hemoglobin and/or red blood cells decreases the ability of the blood to carry oxygen. Symptoms resulting from this are at first subtle. Fatigue, irritability, and loss of appetite are common. As the anemia progresses, compounded by poor intake of iron from the poor appetite, in many instances pallor, severe lassitude, and sometimes fainting result. When the anemia occurs rapidly, as in blood loss due to bleeding or rapid destruction in G-6-PD deficiency, pallor and weakness occur quite dramatically.

Iron-deficiency anemia is, of course, by far the most common anemia, and mercifully the easiest to treat. Simple, inexpensive iron compounds, not the more expensive ones with liver or vitamin B-12, are all that are needed. In a week or two following the prescription of adequate medicinal iron, there is a marked improvement in color, general feeling, state, and appetite.

The other forms of anemia require complex, comprehensive, supportive care, there being no cure in the absolute sense.

Let us reiterate that a sense of general weariness, particularly if accompanied by poor appetite or pallor, requires a medical evaluation and should not be marked off to overwork, alienation, boredom, or depression.

INFECTIOUS MONONUCLEOSIS
(GLANDULER FEVER)

Despite its sobriquet, "the kissing disease," infectious mono, or glandular fever as some call it, is a disease that may be transmitted in a variety of ways, most of which are probably unromantic. Only recently has the probable causative agent, the EB virus (named after Epstein Barr), been associated with it.

This disease can present itself as a severe sore throat or markedly swollen glands, but it can also skip these symptoms and be easily confused with an enervating emotional problem.

It is in most instances not a serious disease, true, but it is bothersome because there is no known specific cure. Its importance is that it can be rather debilitating, and it may involve the liver. Rest and good supportive care are strongly indicated.

There are two little-known complications that on very rare occasions have proved fatal. One is rupture of the spleen; the other is swelling of the structures around the throat and upper airway, which can cause difficulty in breathing. These are rare possibilities, and can readily be prevented by good medical follow-up.

INFECTIOUS HEPATITIS

We have covered this increasingly prevalent disease on page 104. Let us reiterate that it is insidious in onset, and many a victim has been labeled a neurotic by himself or others when indeed he suffered from hepatitis.

The diagnosis is easily made, of course, if the patient turns yellow; but this is not always the case, nor indeed is it always easy to detect. There is at this time no specific cure, but careful medical management is indicated.

URINARY-TRACT INFECTIONS

Careful studies have shown that among the most commonly overlooked infections, particularly in young women, are urinary tract infections. These infections involve our "plumbing": the kidneys, the ureters (tubes leading to the bladder), and the bladder itself. Whereas it is true that there are usually symptoms, pain on urination, frequency of urination, back pain, and fever, none of these need be present. The only indication of a urinary tract infection may be the sense of just not feeling well. Diagnosis is best made by a count of the colonies of bacteria in a urine culture in addition to a microscopic examination of the urine. This type of test should be readily available.

We do not suggest that you tell your doctor what to do, but this condition is so often overlooked and it is so important to know about. We doubt that a concerned physician would mind very much a patient suggesting this possibility to him if she were not feeling well, particularly if she has some of the complaints mentioned above or has had a history of this sort of infection. It should particularly be investigated before childbearing, as severe kidney damage can result if it is overlooked.

HYPOTHYROIDISM

Despite the fact that many signs and symptoms are attributed wrongly to a low thyroid, overweight being the commonest, hypothyroidism or low thyroid state is not rare and may particularly affect the adolescent. The symptoms of hypothyroidism derive from a thyroid hormone deficiency. This hormone helps us create energy from food, helps us grow, and indirectly affects many other bodily functions.

Low thyroid results in fatigue, sluggishness, constipation, and variations in the menstrual cycle. It is only rarely responsible for obesity. In fact, it may cause underweight and poor growth in general. The average obese person is often bigger than his peers, which would not be the case if he suffered from low thyroid. We stress this to counter the general belief that fatness is "glandular," which results at times in unnecessary thyroid medication.

There are laboratory blood tests, the PBI or the T_3 column that easily establish the diagnosis. Treatment is simple: measured replacement of the thyroid hormone.

HYPERTHYROIDISM

In contrast to low thyroid states, there are conditions in which excess thyroid hormone is produced. The symptoms are "nervousness," emotional instability, and weight loss, even in the presence of good or even excessive appetite. Occasionally these symptoms are accompanied by muscular weakness. The thyroid gland in the mid-neck is usually enlarged.

The diagnosis is established with the tests mentioned above, the PBI or the T_3 column, the hormone level in this instance being abnormally high rather than abnormally low.

Treatment depends on drugs such as Propyl Thiouracil or Tapisol that block the production of the excess hormone. Rarely, surgical removal of the enlarged thyroid is necessary.

An enlarged thyroid, like that which is present in hyperthyroidism and sometimes in hypothyroidism, may more commonly appear in an otherwise normal individual around adolescence. A smooth lump just below the Adam's apple may occur without any symptoms. A physician's examination is necessary to rule out other conditions. Often thyroid hormone is prescribed, not because there is insufficient natural hormone, but because it is effective in shutting off the hormone coming from the pituitary that causes the enlargement of the thyroid gland, usually referred to as a goiter.

Rarely, the gland may become inflamed, causing enlargement and pain. This is called "Hashimoto's thyroiditis." It is not serious and can easily be controlled.

TUBERCULOSIS

There was a time in the sixties when it was thought, as it was about venereal disease, that in the United States at least, tuberculosis was close to being eliminated. This unfortunately is not true. Fifty thousand cases are discovered annually, and there are nine thousand deaths each year.

Tuberculosis is more likely to occur in the adolescent than in the adult. Often quiescent childhood forms of it will flare up around adolescence. The reasons for this are far from clear, but in a general sense the stress of adolescent physical development and possibly even the emotional strain may be responsible.

It starts insidiously. The symptoms may be attributed to neurosis. Listlessness, depression, poor appetite, a general feeling of malaise may be experienced. The startling symptoms—coughing, night sweats, fever, and weight loss—are all signs of late stages of the disease.

It is tragic indeed if this disease is allowed to go to such a stage when its detection is so easy and its arrest in the early stages so simple. A yearly tuberculin test, which consists of pricking the arm with a tuberculin-testing needle, is all that is needed. If the test is positive, in two to four days a red, hardened area will appear around the pricked spot.

A positive tuberculin test means that the person has or had the tuberculin germ in him. A chest X-ray will tell more about what state the disease is in. Usually, particularly in adolescence, a specific antituberculous drug is prescribed by mouth for a year, regardless of whether or not active disease is present. This prevents spread of the tuberculous germ and its activation, phenomena more likely to occur in adolescence.

This list of diseases that can be confused with or indeed might mimic emotional disturbances or neuroses is by no means complete, nor was it intended to be. Rather it is a reminder, a warning if you choose, not to neglect symptoms or engage in self-diagnosis. Furthermore, it is clear that a routine yearly physical examination, including a urinalysis, and a yearly tuberculin test is indicated for everyone, but even more so in adolescence, a period of great physiological stress and disease susceptibility.

CHAPTER NINE

Special Care

IMMUNIZATION IN ADOLESCENCE

Immunizations are usually thought of as "shots for tots." They are seldom considered for the adolescent unless he is planning a trip abroad or preparing for camp. Many doctors, as well as parents, are unclear about this subject. This is because the adolescent rarely goes to a doctor for yearly checkups, and he is usually ill when he does go, making him a poor candidate for shots. In addition, many new vaccines are being developed, and the ground rules for administration are still not established. Moreover, research with some of the older vaccines is changing our previously held views about the frequency of boosters. The only point to be made is that it is as important to immunize the adolescent as it is the younger child and infant.

Present recommended schedules:

TETANUS—After the initial series in early childhood, boosters are required only every ten years. Since most children are required to have boosters upon admission to elementary school, a booster is indicated at about fifteen years. *A yearly booster for camp or school is not advisable.*

MUMPS—Males over the age of ten years who have not had mumps should be vaccinated against it to avoid the possibility of sterility from inflammation of the testicles.

GERMAN MEASLES (RUBELLA)—Because of the possible danger of giving this vaccine to a pregnant woman, and because we are not yet certain how long after immunization the fetus can be affected, it is now current practice not to immunize adolescent girls. In individual cases (such as with a mature teen-ager on contraceptives) the physician may appropriately decide to immunize. Techniques are now available for determining the level of naturally acquired immunity to this disease. Such determinations performed on girls at the time of a premarital examination are helpful in deciding the need and timing for vaccination.

POLIO—The oral Sabin vaccine should be administered to any teen-ager who has not been immunized (except for a pregnant one). A booster should be given every four years.

SMALLPOX—The present recommendation is for vaccination every five years.

DIPHTHERIA—This should be given in combination with tetanus immunization every ten years.

WHOOPING COUGH (PERTUSSIS)—This disease is almost unknown in teen-agers. In addition, serious reactions can result from the vaccine in this age group. Therefore, it should not be given.

THE ADOLESCENT AND HIS SKELETON

Posture

The adolescent posture, both moral and physical, is likely to bring him into conflict with the adult world. We will concern ourselves here with straightening up rather than straightening out.

The teen-age boy, particularly if he is long and lean and not heavily muscled (the asthenic type), is prone to slouch. He sits or stands with neck bent, jaw and shoulders forward, and shoulder blades viewed from the back stuck out like wings. It is the antithesis of the military bearing. In and of itself, save for the matter of style, it is not harmful. In years gone by many such young boys were put in braces or corsets to "make them straighten out," all of which, as it turns out, was quite unnecessary.

Exhortations to straighten up are to no avail. The only way to get a boy to correct his posture is to get him to see himself in the mirror or a photograph. Should it turn out then that his silhouette is not to his liking, he may be willing to do something about it.

Should he desire to do so, then exercises designed to increase the tonus of the muscles around the shoulders will help. Any exercise or sport is good, but particularly useful are pushups, carefully graduated weight lifting, and exercise with Indian clubs.

The important thing to remember is that it is not worth nagging anyone about this problem.

The adolescent girl, if she thinks she is too tall, is likely to assume a similar posture. Perhaps some reminder that she is not fooling anybody by slouching, and furthermore it does detract from her appearance, can get her to stand straight, but probably not. Persistent nagging, however, is likely to make her self-conscious, and since bad posture is not really harmful, it is wise not to emphasize it too strongly.

Girls have another kind of postural problem likely to bring them into conflict with their parents. A girl (or, rarely, a boy) may stand swaybacked, exaggerating the hollow of the lower back, the hips and abdomen thrust forward almost to suggest early pregnancy. This will usually get a rise out of parents. This ungainly posture is not in and of itself harmful. It can, however, readily be corrected by strengthening the abdominal muscles.

Sit-ups can help, starting with five per day. The girl should lie flat on her back with hands clasped behind her head. Keeping heels touching the floor, she rises to a sitting position. She should work up gradually to twenty per day. Both the girl and her parents may be surprised at the improvement.

Curvature of the Spine

Curvature of the spine, known to physicians as scoliosis—personally, we like curvature of the spine—is quite common. In a standing position the trunk is tilted one way or other, usually in the region of the chest.

FUNCTIONAL SCOLIOSIS

Most of this curvature is not serious at all and needs no orthopedic correction. It is what is called "functional scoliosis," which means that the curvature is not due to any defect in the spinal column, but rather to the pull of muscles more on one side than another. People who carry books on the right may be noted to tilt to the right, for example. Occasionally, but rarely, if one leg is slightly shorter than another the body will tilt in the same manner.

This can easily be distinguished from more serious structural scoliosis by having the adolescent lean over as if to touch his toes. The back will then straighten out, and no curvature will be seen.

STRUCTURAL SCOLIOSIS OR TRUE CURVATURE OF THE SPINE

The adolescent with true curvature of the spine will not straighten out as he leans forward. Sighting along the back, one can see that the spine is more prominent on one side than the other. The bones stand out more, and the spinal column is fixedly curved.

The cause of this deformity is sometimes difficult to determine. But it is very important to institute corrective procedures as soon as it appears, before the growth spurt that accentuates the deformity. The correction of structural scoliosis requires either special bracing and exercise or, more rarely, a surgical procedure in which the spinal column is straightened out by removal of parts of bone, and casting.

EPIPHYSITIS JUVENILIS OR ROUND BACK

Some rounding of the back is a variation of normal, but there is a more serious situation, rare and not well known but nevertheless important, known as Scheuermann's disease or *Epiphysitis juvenilis*. It is more likely to occur in girls. It may begin with a pain in the back, usually between the shoulders, or it may first be noticed as a deformity. The back becomes rounded, that is, kyphotic.

This is due to an inflammation of the cartilage that lines the adjoining surfaces of the individual rectangular bones that make up the spine, the vertebrae, and requires orthopedic care. It is one more reason that periodic checkups are recommended.

The Limp—Slipped Capital Femoral Epiphysis

There are many ways that adolescents can be self-destructive, but in order not to be accused of complicity, it is wise never to ignore a limp.

I am not here referring to the limp that immediately follows some injury and soon disappears. I am referring to the limp not preceded by injury that persists for days, hopefully not weeks or months, before medical attention is sought.

Adolescents, particularly obese ones, are subject to a condition that if undetected and untreated may result in lifelong misery and deformity. At the head of the great bone of the thigh, the femur, rests the growing end of that bone, the epiphysis, which in adulthood fuses with the rest of the bone. If, however, before this fusion takes place, there should occur slippage of the epiphysis, a hip deformity will result, accompanied by a limp. If pain is present, it may be in the region of the hip or—strangely—the knee. It is important to detect this early before permanent deformity occurs, and it would not be wrong for a boy to suggest to his doctor (he is only human) that the pain he is experiencing in his knee may be coming from trouble in his hip, or that the limp that he may be willing to dismiss as a strain may be indeed a slipped epiphysis.

Osgood Schlatter's Disease

Another way an adolescent may be able to help his doctor is to help him recognize Osgood Schlatter's disease. If he phones him and says, "Hey, Doc [never say Doc], I think I have Osgood Schlatter's disease," he is sure to be impressed, and he is sure to want to see it. The diagnosis is easy. Pain is noted in the leg *below* the knee in the upper portion of the tibia, the major bone of the lower leg. A tender swelling is noticed on that site. Treatment depends on the severity. Since it is self-healing, it can usually be cured by avoiding exercise that involves knee-bending, bicycle riding, basketball, football and other running sports for several months. Swimming and gentle walking are permitted to tolerance. In severe cases casting is sometimes done.

THE NEW-BREAST-OWNER'S MANUAL

So much thought and anticipation precedes the appearance of breasts that after they finally do arrive, the average teen-ager ceases thinking about them. We do not mean to say that one need worry about breasts, but one should remember to pay occasional attention to them. For example, adolescence is the perfect time for a girl to learn and begin the regular nightly practice of self-examination of the breasts. Because cancer of the breast is almost unheard of during the adolescent years, a teen-ager can learn this procedure in an atmosphere devoid of fear. Then when she eventually reaches the cancer-prone years, she will immediately notice even the smallest new bump and be able to bring it to a doctor's attention. The reason breast cancer is so deadly is that most women are too "shy" to examine their breasts and aren't aware of a tumor until it is large enough to see, which is frequently too late.

The Technique of Self-Examination of the Breasts

1. Using the index and third fingers of the opposite hand and starting at the nipple, work your way to the outer edge of the breast tissue, pressing lightly, then deeper as if along the spoke of a wheel.

2. Remember that breast tissue extends up to the collarbone, to the middle of the chest as far as the sternum (breastbone), and well out into the armpit.

3. Start again at the nipple, next to where you began in (1) and repeat.

4. Continue until all breast tissue has been examined in both breasts.

Once you begin regular examinations, you may find that from time to time lumps do appear and that they are usually painful. These are cysts that occur frequently in the two weeks before an expected menstrual period. Cystic stimulation by estrogens and progesterones in the normal course of a month appears to be responsible for the cysts. They tend to occur in older teen-agers, most likely those whose mothers or sisters have the condition called cystic mastitis. They will become smaller and disappear about a month after they come. If they remain longer than that, a doctor should be notified.

The appearance of a discharge from the nipples or a stain on the inside of a bra corresponding to the position of the nipple should be reported to a doctor. While this is a normal occurrence during pregnancy and even for months after delivery of a baby, it may also be the first sign of a condition that requires attention. Hypothyroidism, amenorrhea from a variety of causes, and a tumor of the milk ducts can be associated with a nipple discharge. Some of the tranquilizing drugs can produce both a discharge and amenorrhea, so a girl need not immediately assume she is pregnant if these occur simultaneously.

Selection of a Brassiere

To determine the proper size for your bra take a cloth tape measure and place it on one nipple. Bring it around the broadest part of your back (along the wing bone or scapula) and back around the other nipple to the starting point. Most likely the resultant measurement will be an odd number, and bras always come in even sizes. If that is the case, ask for the next largest size (*e.g.,* if thirty-three, get size thirty-four). In general, breasts that do not sag require an A cup. From there on, the best way to determine the proper cup size is to try the bra on.

Fabric choice is a matter of personal taste. Some of the stretch fabrics occasionally cause an allergic reaction in a sensitive individual, and irritation can result when straps are too tight. We have seen a girl with a black and blue mark and a hard lump in her breast that was found to be the result of pressure from bone in a strapless bra. Perhaps Women's Lib will make these complications obsolete.

HAIR

While baldness on the one hand is a sign of virility, a hairy female is considered unfeminine. This is largely an American phenomenon; the well-dressed European woman with unshaven legs is often shocking to people in this country (women, that is—the men rarely seem to notice).

At puberty, hair on the arms and legs loses its downy appearance and often darkens. In those with familial or ethnic predisposition, the fine hairs above the lip may also darken. These changes are caused by the same factors responsible for acne, namely the increased production of the hormones called androgens. Androgens also cause pubic hair and underarm hair to appear at puberty. Dark hair on the upper lip, on the arms, or even surrounding the areola of the breast is normal in some teen-age females, as it is in males. It is only of concern if the appearance of increased or darkened body hair is accompanied by other changes. If menstruation stops at the same time, it should be investigated. Other associated changes in the female that deserve attention include: deepening of the voice, balding at the temples, enlargement of the clitoris, or a change in the pattern of hair growth in the pubic area so that it grows up toward the navel rather than in the usual triangular area of the pubis. When accompanied by these other symptoms, hirsutism (increased bodily hair) may be an indication of polycystic ovaries, overactivity of the adrenal gland, a tumor of the adrenal gland, or, rarely, an ovarian tumor.

Hirsutism without accompanying symptoms may result from the use of certain drugs. Adrenal hormones are a frequent cause of drug-induced hirsutism. Certain anti-convulsant drugs, namely Dilantin, may also be responsible.

SKIN PROBLEMS

Why is it that junior gets a quarter under his pillow every time he loses a tooth but gets lectures and a trip to the dermatologist with the appearance of each new pimple? This negative attitude toward acne on the part of parents ("He was such a beautiful baby and look at him now!") and the advertising media and the doctors who named it "acne vulgaris" are responsible for much unhappiness among teen-agers today. Actually, getting acne is a very positive event. It means that one is definitely no longer a child. For boys it is a sign of virility, for eunuchs never get acne. For girls it is an outward sign that all the glands responsible for femininity are probably functioning satisfactorily. The oil-secreting glands at the base of the hair roots are target-organs for the sex hormones, just as are the breasts, the voice, and pubic, underarm, and facial hair.

At the time of puberty the walls of these pilose-baceous glands thicken and frequently block the flow of oil or sebum. Oxidation of the sebum in contact with the hair results in a black color, hence the name blackhead for the phenomenon known medically as comedo. The inflammation frequently seen with acne has led to the belief that it is an infection. Recent studies have shown, however, that the bacteria (*Corynebacterium acne* and *Staphylococcus epidermis*) present on the skin of people with acne are also present on the skin of those without it. What is different is the sensitivity of the skin to the fatty acids produced when these bacteria break down the sebum. This response is usually genetically determined, so a good guide to whether an adolescent will have a bad case of acne or not is to ask his parents if they did. The acne lesions can become secondarily infected, which is the rationale for the anti-bacterial soap and antibiotics mentioned below. Antibiotics will also eliminate the bacteria responsible for forming irritating fatty acids.

Status symbol though it may be, there will still be some kids who want to get rid of their acne. For them, the following suggestions are offered:

Treatment of Acne

DIET—Avoid nuts, fish, fried food—particularly the week prior to your expected menstrual period.

HAIR CARE—The scalp tends to be oily in those with acne, and the presence of dandruff can further aggravate the condition. Boys should wash hair each night, and girls, at least twice a week. A shampoo containing sulfur (smells like rotten eggs) is best, *e.g.* Sebulex. Girls should tie their hair back or wear a hair band before going to sleep to prevent hair from coming in contact with the face. The pillow case should be changed or washed frequently.

MAKEUP—What do you do when you know that makeup is bad for acne, yet you must cover up those blemishes? There are medicated creams available for acne sufferers that are flesh-tinted and heal while they cover most blemishes (e.g., Clearasil, Acnomel). They can be used as a makeup base during the day. If these cause irritation, a hypoallergenic makeup base such as that manufactured by Almay is appropriate. Face powder is also made in a hypoallergenic form and should be applied with a new piece of cotton each time. If your nose and chin get shiny during the day and you don't have the opportunity to wash, use a wash-and-dry, followed by a new application of powder. (Throw away the powderpuff in your compact to avoid the temptation to use it—it retains the oils.)

BEARDS—While boys don't have the problem outlined above, they have a similar dilemma. Should they grow a beard to cover the unsightly pimples? While it may temporarily hide them, the presence of a beard makes adequate skin cleansing impossible, and eventually makes the situation even worse.

A DAILY SCHEDULE FOR SKIN CARE
A.M.

a. Wash hands and clean nails with a brush.
b. Wet face and apply a hypoallergenic soap such as Nutrogena with fingers. Work up lather.
c. Rinse.
d. Soak a linen towel in very hot water—then squeeze dry. Apply it to the face. (Facial sauna may substitute.) Pat dry.
e. Apply astringent with clean cotton.
f. Apply medicated cream, such as Clearasil or Acnomel.

P.M.

a. Repeat steps *a* through *e* above.
b. Apply keratolytic lotion (2 percent resorcinol, 3 percent sulfur). Leave on overnight.

It would be helpful to repeat steps *a* through *e* at noontime or when coming home from school. This schedule is calculated to improve your skin dramatically, or if it should prove unsuccessful, at least keep you so busy that you won't have time to brood about your acne.

SUN—Daily sunbaths or sunlamp treatments *in moderation* are helpful.

THE DOCTOR—When pimples are the primary problem, the doctor may prescribe antibiotics (tetracycline) or hormones (estrogens). The reason that teracycline may be useful is that it kills the bacteria that break down the sebum into the irritating fatty acids.

You will notice that no mention is made of limiting the intake of chocolate. This is the result of a recent scientifically controlled study in which teen-agers with mild to moderate acne were given either specially made chocolateless bars or bars containing twice the usual amount of chocolate daily for a total of two months. No significant difference was found in the number of pimples or composition of sebum between the two regimes.

The doctor can remove blackheads effectively and may do so at monthly intervals. Dermabrasion (see Plastic Surgery) or dry-ice treatments may be necessary if scarring is produced, but will have no effect on the pimples or blackheads.

Acne, as we have seen, is basically the result of irritation by certain fatty acids. Scrubbing the skin with a rough washcloth only serves to cause further irritation and aggravate the condition.

Other Common Skin Problems

So-called bath dermatitis is now a well-recognized condition. We have seen it most frequently in the teen-age girl who is self-conscious about increased perspiration, a normal phenomenon in puberty. She embarks on a program of two baths a day, commonly with an antibacterial soap and/or bath powders. These soaps, if used too frequently, cause the protective body oils to be lost, and the bath additives may then cause an irritating or allergic rash. All too often the appearance of a rash prompts the teen-ager to bathe even more and further complicates the problem. The situation can usually be remedied by less frequent bathing and the addition of emollient oils to the bath water.

The adolescent male with "jock itch" can aggravate the condition by too much water and scrubbing too. This condition must be treated with a specific remedy directed at the fungus that caused it.

TEETH

The adolescent is particularly vulnerable to tooth decay. Here are some of the steps one can take to cut down the number of cavities and prevent lifelong dental misery.

1. The teeth should be brushed at least twice a day, but preferably after each meal.
2. It is known that the bacteria responsible for tooth decay need sucrose in order to cause demineralization of enamel. A low-sucrose diet can be very helpful in preventing cavities. An important point to stress is that all sugars are not harmful in this regard, only sucrose. Therefore snacks of popcorn, potato chips, peanuts, fresh fruit, fruit-juices, sugarless gum, and sodas sweetened with saccharin can be substituted for candies, cookies, and regular soda, which contain sucrose.
3. Fluoride mouthwash after each toothbrushing can help to make enamel more resistant to decay.

Adolescence often provides the last chance for correcting problems of "bad bite" as well as some more glaring dental defects that affect appearance. The teen-ager himself is frequently the one to demand dental intervention, thus differing from the younger child who more usually has braces imposed on him. The reasons for this change in attitude are not difficult to understand. At a time when body image is developing, the mouth, the major organ of communication, and the smile, a major determinant of appearance and expression, take on new importance. With improved appearance as the ultimate goal, most teenagers will endure the ordeal of braces. On the other hand, some teen-age girls demand braces as a ready excuse for their pre-existing unpopularity.

The expense of braces makes them a luxury item and in some areas even a status symbol. Nonetheless, in the majority of cases the expense, discomfort, and time invested in orthodontic appliances are compensated for by marked improvement in appearance and health.

The teen-ager with braces must pay meticulous attention to oral hygiene, for cavities flourish where food particles remain in close contact with the teeth, as often happens with braces. A water pick helps to remove these particles without dislodging the braces themselves. Many orthodontists will use fluoride treatments on the teeth about to be braced as protection against decay.

PLASTIC SURGERY

We have spoken about individual differences in appearance, the role of heredity, the process of adjusting to the "new you" that develops during adolescence, and the fact that certain looks are fads and impossible to keep up with when they involve physique. Nevertheless, the teen-ager who discovers that his nickname is Cyrano, Dumbo, Scarface, or Pimple-puss, or is afraid of being called a fag because of his large breasts, will pay no heed to those words of reassurance. Indeed, there are certain circumstances when the most prudent step to take is one that involves changing a bothersome part of one's anatomy. But it is not always justified to say that the mere presence of large features is indication for corrective surgery.

Consider what might have become of Barbara Streisand had her nose been bobbed.

Plastic surgery done on the right person at the right time can be most beneficial. Now, how does one decide who is the right person and when it is the right time? The right person is one who recognizes the defect; who spontaneously expresses a desire for correction, without having been influenced by anyone else (unlike the girl who said she wanted her nose fixed, but on questioning it became clear that it was really her mother who wanted the procedure because the daughter's long nose was a constant reminder of her nose prior to her own surgery); and who has realistic expectations of what surgery can and cannot do. All too often a girl who requests an operation is a case of the White Swan Syndrome (page 29), and expects that she will awaken from surgery a beauty. The well-adjusted adolescent who expects that surgery will change that troublesome feature into one more like that of others in his crowd will be more pleased with its results.

It may be reassuring to know that a survey of girls requesting rhinoplasty (nose bobs) at The Johns Hopkins Hospital showed them to be of above-average intelligence, hard workers in school, and more given to reasoning than their peers. On the other hand, the males wanting this procedure showed a higher incidence of psychopathology.

The timing for surgery is most important. In general most procedures are done when the organ involved has reached its maximal size or has stopped growing. For the nose, this age is generally sixteen years for girls and eighteen years for boys. This will vary from one individual to another, so serial X-rays are generally taken on a yearly basis to determine when growth has stopped. Girls' breasts usually stop growing at about eighteen years of age. Don't forget, however, that after pregnancy breasts are often larger than previously (although we are not suggesting this method for increasing breast size in the adolescent).

Dermabrasion, or planing as a method for minimizing scars of acne, is best done after the adolescent period when the active process itself has stopped.

In general, adolescence is a perfect time for cosmetic surgery because body·image is in the process of formation and such changes can be better integrated into the individual's personality than into that of a static adult.

The procedures most commonly requested by adolescents are rhinoplasty, correction of breasts that are too large or asymmetric (males and females) or too small, dermabrasion for acne scars, and correction of large ears (males more than females).

Rhinoplasty

Whether the problem is one of a broad nose, a long nose, a nose with a hump or a hook, or one with a crooked septum inside, a plastic surgeon can skillfully sculpt it to meet the adolescent's requirements. Remember, however, that he will try to design a nose to fit the face, not that of a fashion model whose picture is brought to his office. After an interview and examination, which will include taking photographs and frequently making plaster impressions, surgery will be scheduled.

In planning for an operation of this kind, a total of five days in the hospital and about another five at home should be allocated. Most teen-agers prefer to schedule surgery during a school vacation, so don't be surprised if the doctor of your choice is booked up far into the future. Even after a date has been set for the operation, the procedure may have to be rescheduled if the hospital doesn't have a bed on the appointed date or if a cold or flare-up of acne makes an operation unwise at that time.

The standard operation, which takes under two hours, is usually done under local anesthesia, which means that the patient will not be asleep but won't feel pain because the nerves to the affected parts of the face will be anesthetized. At the completion of surgery, a splint and bandages are applied to the nose to prevent accidental displacement during sleep. Most are surprised by the lack of pain after rhinoplasty. A common complaint, however, is a dry throat, which results from the need to breathe through the mouth immediately after the operation. The person who thinks he or she will emerge from the bandages a beauty will be shocked to see a rather puffy face with bluish discoloration around the eyes and nose. About three days later, still in this messy state, the patient is usually discharged home to teasing sisters and brothers. The stitches are commonly removed about a week after discharge. While most will be satisfied with the result by the time a month has passed, it is occasionally necessary to perform a second operation called a revision to achieve perfection.

Most plastic surgeons charge between one and two thousand dollars for a rhinoplasty.

Breast Surgery

Breasts may be made larger or smaller by plastic surgery. Because breast tissue doesn't stop growing until about eighteen or nineteen years of age, it is unusual for a doctor to attempt augmentation mammoplasty (enlargement of breasts) prior to this age. The procedure now used by reputable plastic surgeons consists of making a curved incision following the contour of the underside of the breast (which heals into an almost unnoticeable scar) and inserting a soft silicone sac between the breast tissue and the muscle of the chest wall. This operation takes about the same time as a nose bob, but in contrast to that operation, is done while the patient is asleep. A total of about a week is spent in the hospital, followed by approximately a month of restricted use of the arms. The result is a breast that looks entirely normal and feels only slightly harder than natural breast tissue. Augmentation mammoplasty generally costs about one thousand dollars for the surgeon's fee.

The use of the silicone material just described should not be confused with the "silicone injections" used by a few unscrupulous doctors. This method, which doesn't involve an operation, consists of injecting silicone into the breast until the desired size is reached. Unfortunately this size is not maintained, and the breast becomes smaller with time. More significant, however, is the fact that the injection itself may be dangerous if the silicone accidentally enters a blood vessel and gets trapped.

Some girls are bothered by the opposite problem—breasts that are so large that they can't buy a comfortable bra, they feel self-conscious in the company of boys or less-well-endowed friends, and they can't enjoy current styles because of their top-heavy appearance. For them, as well as the occasional boy whose breasts enlarge with the onset of puberty and don't regress within the usual two-year period, surgery may be undertaken to reduce their size (reduction mammoplasty). This is a major operative procedure, and the risks, such as those of general anesthesia and blood loss, must be weighed against the psychological gains of the surgery.

The incision is made underneath the breast, as with the augmentation operation, and the breast tissue removed in part. The nipple is moved upward to approximate the natural position. The incision around the nipple heals so well that it is usually impossible to know that it has been moved. The average hospital stay is one week with restricted use of the arms for about a month thereafter. The surgeon's fee for reduction mammoplasty is generally between one and two thousand dollars.

Dermabrasion for Acne Scars

Plastic surgery is not a cure for acne, but it may be of help to someone whose acne has cleared up leaving scars or deep pits. Dermabrasion, or wire-brush surgery, is the name for the procedure designed to rid the skin of these marks.

The skin is planed with a rotary tool topped with a kind of sandpaper or steel brush, resulting in the formation of a scab. When the scab falls off, the skin beneath is very pink and the pits shallower. Some people, particularly those with heavily pigmented skin, may be made worse by dermabrasion. The procedure itself is done in the doctor's office, and hospitalization is unnecessary, with the usual cost between five and eight hundred dollars.

Ear Flattening

This is a dependable method for improving the appearance of ears that protrude conspicuously. The procedure consists of removing some cartilage, the framework of the ear, through an unnoticeable incision behind the ear. It is usually done under local anesthesia in the hospital and requires only about three days in the hospital. The doctor's fee for this operation is about five hundred dollars.

Crucial to the outcome of any plastic surgery is the ability of the surgeon, but how is one to know this in advance? Your own doctor will usually be able to refer you to someone with a good reputation in the medical community. If there is a medical school in your city, it may be helpful to check with their department of plastic surgery and get the names of those on the faculty. The county medical society can also supply you with a surgeon's name.

In addition to the fees indicated for each operation, usually payable in advance, remember to add the daily cost of hospitalization, operating-room charges, the cost of a prosthesis (*e.g.*, the silicone bag) if required, etc. Also check your hospital insurance policy, for most will not pay for purely cosmetic surgery. For example, if a rhinoplasty is desired to change your appearance, it is not usually covered. If, however, it is performed to correct a crooked (deviated) nasal septum that has interfered with normal breathing, most insurance companies will pay for the operation.

CONTACT LENSES

Even though eyeglasses are currently considered a fashion asset in the mod world, there are still many young people who resent wearing them. For them, contact lenses may be the answer.

There are many advantages to contact lenses. The newer versions that fit over the iris are barely visible, and the larger scleral lenses can be worn while swimming. Those with extreme myopia (nearsightedness) or eyes with unequal refractive power may get better correction and less distortion with contact lenses than with glasses. There is some evidence that myopia may be slowed by contact lenses in the teen-age years. People who do close work with microscopes or ophthalmoscopes are more comfortable with contacts. Peripheral vision is improved by contact lenses, and the risk to an athlete of broken glass injury is nonexistent.

There are also many disadvantages. Not everyone can wear them in comfort, and you cannot tell whether or not you will be able to wear them until after you have paid the still-high price ($150 to $250) for them. Corneal lacerations, usually reversible, can result from their improper use. Lastly, although rarely, one may pop out at a most inopportune time such as while walking down the aisle, as with one girl we know.

Once the decision to try them has been made, the teen-ager should consider the following suggestions:

1. Don't be discouraged if you are not immediately able to perch the tiny lens on your index finger and pop it into your eye. You have spent all your life teaching yourself to blink when a foreign body approaches your eye, and it's going to take a lot of practice to recondition yourself.
2. Keep the lenses and your hands very clean to avoid inflammation of the eye. Always use the

special sterile contact-lens fluid when inserting the lens. Never use plain water, and never, never spit on them. If inflammation does occur, stop using them for a while.

3. Don't use eye makeup for a few weeks, until you have perfected the technique of putting in and taking out the lens and are completely comfortable doing so.

4. If you live in the city (especially New York), wear sunglasses when out of doors. If you don't, you will experience frequent, excruciating bouts of "eye pollution." People who don't wear lenses rarely realize the extent of this problem.

5. Follow your oculist's schedule for building up tolerance.

6. Don't use hair spray or sit under a hair dryer with your lenses in. The former will injure the lenses; the latter may damage the cornea as a result of intense heat.

7. Carry a card saying that you are wearing contact lenses. This may be important in an emergency or accident situation.

ENVIRONMENTAL POLLUTION, TEEN-AGE STYLE

Adolescents chide adults for permitting and contributing to pollution of the environment. Although usually not expressed in quite the same terms, parents of teen-agers with stereo sets also have something to say about who's polluting whose environment. Physiologists in Australia will agree with you. As a result of seeing a number of youngsters who had hearing losses after overexposure to discotheques, Dr. Grahame Clark concluded that the highly amplified, low-pitched sounds of pop music, particularly drums, are harmful over a long period of time. He found that the noise level in discotheques was about one hundred decibels or ten to fifteen decibels higher than a safe level for continuous exposure. Damage to the cochlea was found in adolescents who had attended discotheques once or twice a week for about six to twelve months.

Further studies on this subject by Dr. Frederick Day showed that this hearing damage occurred insidiously and that susceptibility varied from individual to individual. He showed that 16 percent of subjects who listened to music at 110 decibels had permanent hearing loss. Moreover, he found that pain was not a good indication of damage.

We do not know whether this information will cause the teen-ager to turn down his record player or not, but at least he should know about it.

ATHLETICS AND THE ADOLESCENT

Physical activity should be part of the life style of the adolescent. No less important than the cultivation and stimulation of the mind is the development of a healthy body. Adolescence is probably a crucial time for regular physical exercise, for evidence is accumulating that the beneficial effects are both immediate and far-reaching. The immediate benefits are a sense of well being and general better health. Less well known is the fact that physical exercise results in increased height and some decrease in hip width.

Heart attacks, so devastating to the middle-aged American male and increasing in the female, may indeed be prevented by exercise in adolescence. Here is how it works. The blood vessels that supply the heart, the coronary arteries, can often be made more effective during adolescence under the influence of various hormones and consistent physical exercise. The blood supply not only to the heart but to all the organs of the body can be enriched by exercise in youth. Thus not only heart attacks but strokes may be thwarted by an adolescent concern with athletics.

We have stressed the importance of physical activity in the prevention of obesity. (A table of calorie expenditure for various activities is provided on p. 40).

There can be an athletic program for everyone, no matter what his physical status. Prior to starting the program, everyone should have a physical exam. We stress this because one often hears, "I feel well. What do I have to see the doctor for?"

Here are some of the reasons.

HIGH BLOOD PRESSURE

A teen-ager with high blood pressure may feel perfectly well.

We have often seen high blood pressure discovered in a routine physical exam. Undetected high blood pressure and vigorous physical exercise may result in sudden death in several ways.

High blood pressure due to a narrowing of the aorta, the great vessel that carries the blood from the left side of the heart, can now be easily corrected surgically. If undetected, brain hemorrhage can result, particularly after vigorous exercise.

High blood pressure due to kidney diseases of various sorts may be similarly disastrous. Let us stress that in all instances, the victim has *no* symptoms.

HEART MURMURS

Heart murmurs are usually not a sign of any disease. The vast majority of them are "innocent," but a physician will have to decide. Aortic stenosis, which causes a characteristic murmur, may result in sudden death after vigorous exercise.

Less dramatic, but important to check before athletic programs are undertaken, are the presence of a history of head injuries, convulsions, asthma, heart disease, anemia, etc.

An athletic program, however, can be adapted to anyone. There is, happily, much more awareness of this, and athletic programs are no longer just for the "jocks." Athletic activity is of equal importance for girls and boys.

Some General Problems Arising from Athletics

HEAT STROKE

Heat stroke occurs when the sweating mechanism is ineffective in lowering body temperature. The victim collapses; his skin is dry and warm.

He should be cooled immediately with cool water—if possible, immersed in a cool tub with his head carefully supported to prevent drowning. Get immediate medical attention.

HEAT EXHAUSTION

Heat exhaustion causes weakness or faintness and profuse sweating. There is, in the course of exercise, loss of water plus salt. The salts are predominantly sodium, but there is loss of potassium too. Salt tablets with the amount of water usually recommended on the bottle should be administered. There are now commercial beverages available, favored by coaches, that are quite good in preventing heat exhaustion if drunk before and after exercise. Adequate amounts of any fluids containing sodium and potassium can be used to prevent heat exhaustion. We offer our own formula. It is tasty and inexpensive, and not only can prevent heat exhaustion but has markedly cut down fatigue as well.

Make up a quart of frozen lemonade as per directions on the can. It is usually four and one-third cans of water to the can of concentrate. Add to this three grams of sodium chloride in the form of three one-gram salt tablets. The lemonade contains potassium, so only the sodium chloride should be added; avoid the tablets that contain sodium and potassium. Ice the lemonade. Drink liberally before exercise and weigh yourself before and after activity. Any weight loss you notice will be primarily salt and water. Two pounds is equivalent to about a quart of the solution. By replacing the loss with a balanced salt solution, heat exhaustion, cramps, and fatigue can be sharply reduced.

Injuries

HEAD INJURIES

An injury to the head should always be respected and false heroics avoided. If a blow to the head is sustained and there is any dizziness or unconsciousness, however brief, the person must be made to stop whatever he is doing immediately. Unconsciousness, incoordination, clumsiness, amnesia from the injury call for immediate medical examination and observation.

ABDOMINAL INJURIES

Blows to the abdomen should never be taken lightly. They may cause damage to a series of nerves to the coeliac plexus, resulting in immediate sweating, pallor, and occasional collapse. Or the spleen, on the upper left side of the body, may be injured or ruptured, immediately producing severe pain and then collapse. Injuries to the liver, on the upper right side, which are less common, may do the same. Injuries to the pancreas may produce abdominal pain and vomiting. Injuries to the kidney, usually from being hit in the back, cause pain and blood in the urine.

Injuries to the testicle can cause acute swelling and pain similar to and sometimes indistinguishable from torsion of the testes (see p. 72).

We are not attempting to provide the reader with a means of diagnosing abdominal injuries, but rather to persuade him to take them seriously and obtain immediate medical care.

STRAIN

A strain is inflammation of a muscle because of misuse. It occurs commonly in the thighs or calves.

SPRAIN

Sprain is the wrenching of a joint producing stretching or laceration of the ligaments. It usually occurs at the knee or ankle.

All weight should be removed from the affected limb, an ice pack applied, and of course, medical attention sought.

FRACTURE

If fracture of the back or neck is suspected because of pain or inability to move, the person should not be moved until proper medical supervision and a stretcher are available. Arms or legs where fracture is suspected should be immobilized with a splint that extends from the joint below the injury to prevent movement of the bone. Immediate medical attention is required.

CRAMP

Occasionally as a result of heat exhaustion, sometimes for other reasons, one can experience a muscle cramp. They are usually in the calf muscle. A ball-like "knot" of muscle in the calf is felt. Lying down on the back and having someone pull back on the foot so as to counteract the contraction of the calf muscle is very helpful for relieving specific pain and spasm. Follow with warm, wet compresses or a heating pad. Take plenty of fluids. See the special formula for heat exhaustion on p. 141.

BLISTERS

Blisters are due to friction. Large blisters should be opened with a sterilized needle (made red hot in a flame), dressed with an antiseptic cream, and bandaged.

Specific Sports and Safeguards

BASEBALL

The need for proper headgear is obvious.

PITCHING

Due to the fact that the growing ends of the bones, the epiphyses, have not yet united with the shaft of the bones in the teen-ager, they are readily susceptible to injury. If injured, they can cause growth arrest in the bone affected with the end result of a shorter arm. A boy of fourteen or less who attempts to pitch a curve or screw ball may injure the epiphyses and cause permanent damage. Therefore no one under fourteen should do so.

FOOTBALL

Carefully check equipment to prevent head and body injuries. The knees can easily be injured in football by fast pivoting or being hit from the side or behind. Injuries to the ligaments around the knee or to the epiphyses should be watched for. Adolescents of thirteen to sixteen, at least, should play with careful supervision, if at all.

CHAPTER 10

Special Problems

TEEN-AGE SMOKING

The following is an analysis of a report by the American Cancer Society evaluating adolescents' attitudes toward smoking.

1. Smoking is a major cause of cancer of the lung.
2. Smoking significantly increases one's chances of having a heart attack in later years.
3. Women who smoke regularly during pregnancy have smaller babies than those who are not smokers. Since the size of a newborn influences his chances for survival, infants of smokers are at a disadvantage.
4. Smoking decreases your ability to breathe. This is not a long-range effect. As few as ten puffs of cigarette smoke will reduce airway conductance of the lungs by 50 percent, and this deleterious effect will last for an hour in either the one-time or chronic smoker, regardless of age. Oxygen intake is limited as a result, and this causes, in turn, diminished endurance. It should then be apparent why smoking is forbidden for athletes.
5. According to the American Cancer Society, in the past two years the percentage of teen-age smokers in this country rose an average of 4 percent. The percentage of twelve-year-old-boy smokers doubled in that same period of time.
6. Twelve percent of girls and almost 19 percent of boys in the twelve-to-eighteen-year range are regular smokers.

7. In the same two-year period the number of adult smokers decreased by four to six million.

8. Almost three-quarters of the fifteen hundred teen-agers interviewed in the Cancer Society study believed that smoking caused cancer, including the 65 percent who themselves smoked.

9. Teen-agers are 100 percent more likely to smoke if their siblings and friends smoke and 50 percent are more apt to if the adults they know do so.

10. Teen-age smokers were reportedly more nervous, more anxious, more anti-establishment than non-smokers. They were also poorer students.

11. Younger teen-agers smoked for "social" reasons, primarily to look older, and older teens claimed to smoke to relieve "tension."

12. Most adult smokers began their smoking in the teen-age years.

These findings confirm what we've always suspected, namely that in spite of knowing of the dangers, teen-agers will continue to smoke, primarily because of social pressures. The situation has not been helped by advertisements that portrayed male smokers as young, virile, and handsome and the girls as beautiful, carefree, sexy, and above all, healthy. Because teen-agers tend to identify with these models, our plan is to reduce teen-age smoking by the negative use of the capacity to identify, as in the following hypothetical TV advertisement:

The tiny screen is filled with the picture of an old hobo. He is sickly looking, dirty and unkempt. He is wearing oversized clothes as if he had lost weight. His skin and teeth are yellow. He appears cachectic and consumptive. He is puffing on a cigarette, and as he finishes he says, "I'd walk a mile for a Camel."

Although it might raise objections from the United Hobos of America, it might get a lot of teen-agers to quit smoking.

BED-WETTING

Bed-wetting, or enuresis, is the inability to maintain bladder control during sleep. When control has never been achieved, it is called primary enuresis. This is more than likely a developmental problem, representing an immaturity of the bladder-control mechanism. With time children with primary enuresis improve, but it is by no means rare to find an adolescent or even a young adult with bed-wetting problems.

Before primary enuresis can be treated, all organic causes must be ruled out. The physician will want to know if there is any trouble with urination during the day. For example, does straining occur during urination? Is there pain? Is there dribbling? Is there a history of urinary-tract infection or symptoms of the same? He will want to do some tests: a urinalysis to measure the specific gravity of the urine (can the kidneys concentrate the urine to prevent excessive urination?) and to detect the presence of sugar, indicating diabetes; a microscopic examination to search for pus cells or red blood cells indicating infection or kidney disease; a culture of the urine to rule out infection more certainly. If all of these plus a careful physical examination are unrevealing, the physician may want to do X-rays of the kidney and the bladder.

Radio opaque material is inserted into the bladder by means of a catheter. This enables the X-ray to show bladder size and shape as well as any abnormalities in the bladder outlet, the tube called the urethra that leads directly to an opening in the female and into the penis in the male. Dye is then injected into the veins to outline the kidney structure. All of this may sound complicated, but it is actually simple and painless and does not require hospitalization. Should all of these tests prove to be negative, as they usually do, then we can be assured there is no "disease" in the structures causing the problem.

The cause may be small bladder capacity. There are individuals who cannot hold a large enough volume of urine in their bladders to get through the night. This may or may not be apparent on the X-rays; but if a child is constantly running to the bathroom during the day, there is reason to be suspicious. The average teen-ager has to void about five to seven times per day.

If small bladder capacity is suspected, there are bladder-stretching procedures. First, rather than restricting fluids, fluids should be encouraged. An attempt should be made to hold in the urine until it becomes painful. Drugs may be helpful. Occasionally the use of tincture of belladonna, a drug that relaxes the smooth musculature in the bladder wall and in addition tightens the sphincter, which allows urine to pass out of the bladder, is helpful in increasing bladder capacity. We usually start out with five drops three times a day, increasing by one drop each day up to fifteen drops three times a day. This is ordinarily continued for several months. If excessive dryness of the mouth or flushing of the skin is noticed, the dose is dropped back to the next lower dose. This, of course, should be done only under the supervision of a physician.

A more recent drug with the generic name of imipramine hydrochloride has proven to be successful in about two-thirds of the cases in which it has been used. It can be employed either in cases of suspected small bladder capacity or in any case of primary enuresis in which no structural disease has been found. Although it is a mood elevator, an antidepressant, it also acts much like belladonna, and in addition, affects levels of sleep. It seems to reduce the number of times per night that sleep levels change from deeper to lighter. Bed-wetting and also probably sleepwalking (somnambulism) are now believed to be disorders of arousal occurring during these sleep-level changes.

Imipramine's major effects seem to be in most instances independent of its effect on emotions. The drug, if successful over a period of three months, is discontinued. The enuresis in most instances remains improved in terms of number of accidents.

What about emotional problems?

Only rarely is primary enuresis the result of emotional problems and susceptible to treatment by psychotherapy. In the vast majority of cases it is a developmental problem, much like a delay in walking or talking or singing on key.

We have stressed primary enuresis. What about secondary enuresis, the appearance of bed-wetting in a previously controlled person? This is very rare in teen-agers, and when it does occur, one must suspect and investigate such causes as diabetes or infection, both of which lead to frequent urination.

It is rare indeed to have a teen-ager start bed-wetting for emotional reasons, but if all organic causes have been ruled out, psychiatric evaluation should be undertaken. There is a curious association between fire-setting and bed-wetting, and the former tendency should be looked for. The two tendencies existing together indicate a serious emotional problem and immediate psychiatric aid is called for.

DRUGS

Two British psychiatrists who believed that the only one who could tell a "junkie" is another "junkie" devised a questionnaire for teen-age heroin users to determine their criteria for detecting drug use in another teen-ager. They also asked the same questions of parents of known drug users. The parents and their offspring agreed on most points, with two exceptions. While the parents rated "inability to concentrate" high on their list, the teen-agers rarely were aware of this problem. Conversely, the kids noted that someone on drugs repeatedly looks down at the site of his last needle puncture. Parents never picked this up. From the answers of the drug-using adolescents and their parents the following composite picture is compiled: The drug user is withdrawn, wants to be left alone, frequently refuses food, shuns noise and bright lights, does poorly in school, receives many phone calls, and leaves the house frequently.

Pause and consider how much of what they said can describe any teen-ager in love.

The question "How can I tell if my teen-ager is using drugs?" can be answered, but let's ask if it should be. To arm parents with the tools of drug detection is to convert them into law-enforcement officers. They can become adversaries of the very people they are struggling so hard to keep from losing. What is accomplished if by searching his or her room, pills or pot are found, of if he is brought to the doctor's office for a "drug test"? To "find out" under such circumstances will only serve to drive a wedge between parents and teen-agers. Only the symptom will be uncovered, not the cause for it.

We have found that the best way to discover if someone is using drugs is to ask him. A family in which the parent can come and ask out of honest interest rather than in an effort to "get something" on his child is the family in which the kid will also answer honestly. If the answer if affirmative, a rational dialogue, based on mutual respect, can be established and a common solution sought. The first step toward achieving this utopian situation is education of both parties concerning the effects and dangers of all drugs. One thing that precludes a meaningful discussion between kids and their parents about drugs is a parent who speaks authoritatively on a subject about which he knows little but feels a lot. Another thing that results in the same impasse is the teen-ager who, although sounding more expert, has derived all his knowledge from his probably equally uninformed peers.

The following is an attempt to present what is known at the present time about the drugs commonly used by today's teenagers. It is based on medical literature as well as personal experience with the medical care of three thousand adolescent drug users over the past two years. One-half of this group were heroin users. Glue-sniffers made up one-quarter of this New York City-based population. The remaining group of approximately seven hundred consisted of teen-agers who took amphetamines, barbiturates, and hallucinogens such as LSD and marijuana. Five percent required hospitalization as the result of their drug use, and five died while hospitalized.

Marijuana (Pot, Grass, Mary Jane, Reefers, Joints)

Marijuana is produced from the resin in the flowering parts and high leaves, as well as the recently fertilized ovary and unripened fruit of the female plant *Cannabis sativa*. This plant, also a source of hemp fiber and seed oil, grows in temperate and hot, dry areas, and flourishes in human excrement. Those political murderers in Asia Minor in the thirteenth century A.D. who smoked the pure resin of the plant, called hashish, were called hashishins, from which comes the word "assassin." Cannabis resin has been found to contain a variety of constituents, including cannabidiolic acid, cannabichromene, and delta-1-tetrahydrocannabinol. The former two have been found to have sedative properties. The hallucinogenic effects of marijuana appear to reside in the delta-1-tetrahydrocannabinol fraction, which has recently been synthesized in the laboratory. The pure synthetic form is a potent hallucinogen, even more so than LSD. Recent studies, published in their preliminary form, indicate that when tetrahydrocannabinol (THC) is given to pregnant rabbits it can pass into the placenta, and indeed is found in higher concentrations there than in the blood of the mother animal. "So what?" you may ask. The importance of this finding is that an earlier experiment with cannabis resin in mice showed that it could produce serious birth defects when injected into the abdomen of a pregnant animal. A legitimate criticism of this experiment was that the resin was introduced into the amniotic fluid of the fetus and that there was no proof that the substance could pass into the fetus naturally. The rabbit experiment suggests that at least in one animal the pure THC can indeed pass into the placenta and possibly harm the fetus.

When presented with experimental data such as this, teen-agers are usually justifiably critical. A mouse is not a human, and smoking pot probably doesn't result in such a high blood level of cannabis extract as in the experiments, they will say. They are right as far as they go, but we should recall that the link between smoking and lung cancer in humans was first realized when Dr. Ernst Wynder and his associates painted an extract of cigarette smoke on the skin of rats and produced a skin cancer. Critics then said the same thing: a rat is not human and the dose of extract is probably higher than that which results from smoking cigarettes.

It may also be salient to mention that the FDA recently removed cyclamates from the market on even weaker evidence.

"Marijuana has been used for thousands of years. If it were harmful, we would have known about it before now," is a common statement by knowledgeable teen-agers. The ancient Oriental cultures in which its use was heavy were the same ones in which there was a high rate of infant mortality and poor life expectancy. Certainly nutritional and infectious factors, rather than hash, mainly- were responsible, but we have no way of knowing to what extent if any the use of marijuana contributed to this. It is only in recent history that we have been aware and able to study potential chromosomal, tumor-producing, and biochemical effects.

Another fact that is frequently lost sight of is that until recently only men smoked marijuana, so that even if it could cause birth defects we would not have known it until now when both girls and boys are smoking pot.

Recall that more than a half-century passed while

people smoked cigarettes thinking they were harmless. Rather than dwell on this point, suffice it to say that research into the effects of marijuana is just beginning. It is possible that it will be found to have no adverse physical effects, but right now we don't know that, and it is irresponsible for scientists to say that it is harmless until more is known. Thus far the little that is known about it scientifically seems to point in the other direction.

Many enlightened teen-age girls have told us that they will not risk any drug because of the possibility that it will eventually be found to cause birth defects. Indeed, it is an axiom in the new drug subculture that one should not use any drug or even smoke pot when pregnant. What these girls do not know is that all the eggs that will ultimately be released from the ovary during a lifetime are present, albeit in an immature form, when a female is born. As a result, a substance that affects chromosomes can act on the egg before it is fertilized and potentially can be harmful even if taken years before pregnancy. The other, more obvious problem is that a girl doesn't usually know she is pregnant until most of the fetus' development has taken place, and a harmful substance is much more potent when taken early in pregnancy.

Today's teen-agers smoke marijuana in "joints," cigarettes that are made by rolling the crushed leaves and flowers in papers available in most stores selling psychedelia. Hashish, the form of cannabis that has about eight times the potency of marijuana, is smoked in a pipe. According to sociologist Erich Goode, who studied the marketing of marijuana recently, the retail price of a joint is between fifty cents and one dollar. He also found, however, that almost no one buys an individual joint, but rather a small bulk quantity from which he rolls his own. A "nickle bag" sells for five dollars and contains between one-eighth and one-fourth of an ounce, which is enough to make between eight and twelve cigarettes. Another interesting find of his was that in contrast to the marketing of heroin, which involves mainly non-drug-using pushers, most selling of marijuana is done by users. Indeed, nearly half of his informants had sold at least once.

The odor of marijuana is distinctive and resembles that of burning rope. Because of this most pot smokers burn incense to disguise the odor.

Routine tests for detection of marijuana in the urine are not available.

Just how extensive is marijuana smoking? Because of the fact that it is illegal, it is very difficult to know for sure. In the spring of 1969 a Gallup poll found that one-quarter of American college students had tried marijuana at least once. In January of 1970 a newspaper reported that 50 percent of the almost seven hundred Amherst students who answered a questionnaire had smoked pot occasionally and that 10 percent used it more than twice a week. In our own survey of adolescents between the ages of thirteen and nineteen who were admitted to our in-patient service for medical or surgical problems, 5 percent who answered a questionnaire admitted to marijuana use.

The first studies done on marijuana under controlled conditions were reported by Drs. Weil, Zinberg, and Nelson at the end of 1968. On the basis of their studies the following physiologic effects of marijuana on humans are finally established:

1. Heart rate is increased by marijuana in both new users and chronic users. This effect is maximal fifteen minutes after smoking.
2. Respiratory rate is unchanged by marijuana in new users. In chronic users there is a small but statistically significant increase in respiratory rate.
3. The size of pupils is unaffected by marijuana.
4. Marijuana causes dilation of the blood vessels of the conjunctiva, the protective membrane over the whites of the eyes. As a result the eyes of a pot smoker appear reddened within an hour after smoking.

5. Blood sugar is not lowered by marijuana. This was previously considered to be the cause of the voracious appetite of most pot smokers, which remains unexplained.

Other than the subjective reports of marijuana users who report feelings of hilarity, euphoria, and excitation, and occasionally hallucinations, little has been known until recently about the effect of the substance on the mind. Dr. Weil and his associates have shown, on the basis of psychological testing under controlled conditions, that marijuana in doses usually smoked by young people today has no effect on the subject's capacity for sustained attention. Those smoking it for the first time did demonstrate impaired performance on simple intellectual and psychomotor tests—and the higher the dose the greater the impairment—but regular users showed no impairment. All psychologic effects were greatest within one half hour of smoking and had completely disappeared within three hours. In more recent experiments, these same researchers showed that understanding was not impaired by marijuana but that immediate memory was significantly interfered with. As a result speech was affected to the extent that people using marijuana frequently forget what they were about to say next and had a tendency to go off on tangents because they would lose their line of thought.

Psychological tests are one thing, but what about real-life situations? There has been much understandable concern about the possible risks of driving while under the influence of marijuana. Investigators at the Department of Motor Vehicles of the State of Washington compared the effects of marijuana and alcohol on simulated driving performance in experienced smokers under controlled conditions. Interestingly, they found that those experiencing a marijuana high accumulated more speedometer errors than under drug-free conditions, but that there were no significant differences in accelerator, brake, signal, and total errors than under normal conditions. Obviously, more research of this kind is needed and under way.

The psychiatric literature is rapidly filling with reports of marijuana-induced psychoses. The factors responsible are difficult to sort out and probably relate to pre-marijuana personalities and stress situations. There is, however, one pattern that appears to be emerging with great frequency in chronic users. It has been referred to as the "amotivational syndrome," but we prefer to call it the "anti-Horatio Alger syndrome." It is the pattern of subtle change from the achievement-oriented behavior of middle-class students into passivity and lack of goal direction, commonly called "dropping out." Kids may argue that they are shunning the hypocritical, materialistic society of their elders and that pot is just part of their style rather than the cause of their dropping out. It is possible that the same variables are responsible for both, rather than cause and effect, but nonetheless, this pattern is seen in regular rather than occasional users.

Most critics of marijuana feel that its danger lies in its potential for leading to abuse of heroin and other "hard" drugs. It has been stated that 80 percent of heroin users had first smoked pot. While this may or may not be true in the population questioned, it is equally true that many more experiment with pot and never go on to use heroin. It has been our experience with a ghetto population in New York that most heroin users had their first contact with hallucinogenic agents in the form of glue rather than pot. The issue should really not be which is more likely to lead to harder drugs, but rather, what is the end result of any substance abuse by adolescents. It is one thing for an adult, whose attitudes and approach to life are already formed, to get high on alcohol or pot at a party, and another for an adolescent to repeatedly seek any toxin for the purpose of escaping from reality as the alternative to solving a problem. It is in adolescence that the pattern of problem solving must be established. To avoid problems by "turning on" as a teen-ager is to become an adult who may not be able to deal with frustration constructively.

Heroin (H, Horse, Skagg, Stuff)

While the effects of marijuana are still being studied, those of heroin are well known. Heroin is derived from opium, the milky juice of unripe seed capsules of the poppy plant grown in Asia Minor. Opium, known to man before recorded history, has been used since the third century B.C. to control diarrhea and alleviate pain. It was not until the nineteenth century that crude opium was purified and its active ingredients—morphine, codeine, and papverine—isolated. Of these, morphine is responsible for the pain-killing and euphorogenic properties of the parent compound. Through substitution of two components of the morphine molecule by a chemical procedure termed acetylation, it is transformed into heroin, more potent than either morphine or opium as a pain killer, mood elevator, and depressant to breathing. Because of its potency as a respiratory depressant, as well as its addictive properties, heroin has been removed from the druggist's shelf and can no longer be prescribed as a pain killer by physicians in the United States. Nonetheless, heroin users number in the hundred thousands, the exact number impossible to determine.

The teen-age heroin user was almost unknown before the 1960s. In 1964 the New York City Narcotics Register of The Department of Health began and listed 7 percent of heroin addicts as under twenty years of age. By 1968 this percentage had doubled. It is obvious that these figures represent the peak of the iceberg and that most heroin users are not systematically reported. Extrapolating from the number of deaths from heroin use in New York City, the Chief Medical Examiner's Office estimates that there are currently 25,000 teen-age heroin users. Our own experience with a population of teen-agers detained by the courts shows that the twelve-year-old heroin user is unfortunately no longer a rarity.

The teen-ager is usually introduced to heroin by a "friend," who may urge him to snort (inhale) some of the white powder to get high. By this method of administration, the full effect of the heroin is appreciated about a half hour later. Curiously, the predominant effect is an unpleasant one, as described by Claude Brown in *Manchild in the Promised Land:*

> Everything was getting rosy, beautiful. The sun got brighter in the sky, and the whole day lit up and was twice as bright as before. . . . Everything was so slo-o-o-w. And then my head started. My head seemed to stretch, and I thought my brain was going to burst. It was like a headache taking place all over the head at once and trying to break its way out. And then it seemed to get hot and hot and hot. . . . I tried to get up, but my legs were like weights. I got scared. I'd never felt this way in my life before. . . . My guts felt like they were going to come out. Everything was bursting out all at once, and there was nothing I could do. It was my stomach and my brain. My stomach was pulling my brain down into it, and my brain was going to pull my guts out and into my head. And I said, "O Lawd, if you'll just give me one more chance, . . . I'll never get high again." And then it seemed like everything in me all of a sudden just came out, and I vomited. . . . I thought we'd just killed ourselves.

For some macabre reason, these devastating effects of the first encounters with heroin do not usually serve as deterrents to future use in the pursuit of euphoria.

Those who desire a more immediate high or who find that they soon need more heroin for a high than they can comfortably inhale at any one time usually graduate to skin-popping, the practice of injecting heroin, mixed and heated with water, into the skin to form a button-like swelling. According to the teen-age users, a high is achieved within fifteen minutes by this method. Many continue to skin-pop indefinitely, while a smaller number go on to inject the heroin directly into a vein, called "mainlining," to get high instantaneously.

Addiction may result from heroin use by any of the three routes of administration, although there is much individual variation as to the amount, frequency, and duration of use necessary for this to occur. In general, however, anyone who uses heroin on a daily basis for more than a month is likely to become physically addicted to the substance. Psychological addiction is more difficult to predict and measure and probably occurs sooner. A person is considered physically addicted if he demonstrates characteristic changes such as dilated pupils, running nose, yawning, restlessness, muscle cramps, "gooseflesh," stomach cramps, diarrhea, elevated blood pressure, and convulsions or shock when deprived of his drug.

The heroin user continually walks the tightrope between the constantly increasing dose necessary to get a high and that which may cause death, the so-called overdose.

Heroin has an affect on nearly every bodily system. At the level of the central nervous system it acts to kill pain, and as a result, the heroin user may be unaware of conditions heralded by this symptom. For example, a study of ex-addicts found a large proportion of them to have stomach ulcers. In retrospect, most had had no pain while on heroin and had misinterpreted their ulcer pain as withdrawal symptoms when off the drug.

It has already been noted that heroin has a powerful depressant effect on breathing. In addition, it serves to inhibit the cough reflex. While this may be an advantage to someone with a cold, it removes an important defense mechanism. Aspiration pneumonia (pneumonia caused by fluid or food going down the wrong "pipe") and possibly death, can result. The finding of an increased incidence of tuberculosis in adult heroin users is more likely a result of their generally poor nutrition, as this disease does not appear commonly in the adolescent heroin user. All people who die from an "overdose" of heroin are found to have fluid in their lungs. Some of our patients developed asthma while on heroin which disappeared after they discontinued it. Consequently, it is possible that allergy, either to the heroin or something with which it is mixed, plays some role in its effect on some users.

The effect of heroin on the endocrine system has been demonstrated in animals and humans as well. It has been shown to interfere with the functioning of the master gland, the pituitary. It is in adolescence that the endocrine system undergoes its greatest change. It should not be surprising, then, that the introduction of a drug during this crucial time of life has profound consequences. While heroin is capable of producing a variety of menstrual irregularities in some adult women, we have found that fully one-third of teen-age girls using heroin stop menstruating altogether. That most do not resume menstruation for months following cessation of use may indicate long-lasting effects and possibly sterility in teen-agers whose cycles have not had a chance to become regulated.

Ulcers are not the only result of heroin's action on the gastrointestinal tract. Every heroin user, regardless of age, experiences constipation as a consequence of the drug's ability to slow the wavelike contractions of the intestine. This same effect on the bladder muscle results in infrequent urination.

A recent report of structural changes seen with the electron microscope in the livers of heroin users with hepatitis reopens the controversy about a possible direct effect of the drug. Indeed the teen-age heroin users whom we have treated for hepatitis differ from non-drug-using adolescents with the same disease in that they take longer to improve and many appear to be headed toward cirrhosis or chronic impairment of the liver ending with liver failure and death.

Were heroin legal and available in the pure state, the user would still be subject to these effects. That it is not legal and is mixed with a variety of fillers poses additional threats to him.

Because it is illegal, the user has none of the guarantees of quality control and safety that accompany licensed drugs. As a result, a five-dollar bag of heroin (they usually cost between two and ten dollars a bag) may on one day contain one milligram of heroin and on the next, fifteen. Most "overdose" deaths are caused by this phenomenon.

In order to make more money from their heroin supply, dealers mix it with milk sugar, which resembles the white powder of the original material. The heroin user is aware of this "cutting" and usually tastes it before buying. If sweet, it is rejected. If bitter, it is accepted as "good stuff." The name of the game, then, is to add bitter substances to the heroin-sugar mixture. Quinine, the old popular one, is now in short supply because of its diversion to Vietnam for prevention and treatment of malaria. The quest now is to find substitutes. We have seen everything from antihistamines to local anesthetics added for this purpose. Indeed, one teen-age girl addict recently interviewed by the press claimed to have added roach powder because it was all she could find. An epidemic of tetanus was once traced to spores that had settled on a dusty table on which a heroin dealer cut and packaged the drug.

To the dangers imposed by the pharmacologic properties of heroin and those resulting from its unscrupulous preparation, add those related to the method of its administration. When "snorted" or administered by nasal inhalation, it can result in irritation of the mucous membrane, or in rare instances in perforation of the septum, leaving a large hole in the cartilage that separates the two nostrils. When skin-popped, it frequently causes abscesses. These can then provide a source of generalized infection. More importantly, these abscesses make an excellent breeding place for tetanus germs, and tetanus or lockjaw is now one of the most dreaded complications of this mode of administration. Mainlining can result in foreign matter in the bloodstream. This can lodge in the lungs and cause abscesses there. Infection of the valves of the heart is another complication of this practice. The use of an unsterilized needle for either skin-popping or mainlining is often followed weeks or months later by hepatitis (see pages 104-107).

Heroin can interfere with health in still another way. Attempts at concealment of the drug have been known to have dire consequences. One man who came to the operating table for obstruction of the intestine was found at surgery to have a condom filled with heroin as the cause of obstruction. He had swallowed it with the hope of reclaiming it days later in the toilet. The same mode of concealment has also been associated with "overdose" death from sudden release of the condom's contents when it broke after being swallowed.

The dangers of heroin use are well known to the addicts, for all have had friends die from one of them, but the horrors of withdrawal symptoms, coupled with the teen-ager's feeling of indestructibility, are sufficient deterrent to stopping. Moreover, for the dropout, the daily cycle of "shooting," the "rush" that follows, the euphoria and "nodding," and the eventual scramble to make connections for getting money and then more stuff to start all over again gives a structure and purpose to an otherwise empty existence. One ghetto teen-ager said, "When I buy good stuff, I'm somebody important. The kids tell me, 'Man, you know where to get it good.' "

Heroin use can be suspected in an individual who has small pupils, who is tired all the time, who has needle tracks or marks, or who has abscesses and bumps on his skin where heroin is "popped." The mucous membranes of the nose are reddened from inhalation of heroin or cocaine, but really this looks very much the same as the nose of someone with a mild cold or allergy.

If heroin has been used, it can be detected in the urine, as morphine, up to forty-eight hours after the last dose. Quinine, which, as we have seen, is frequently added to the heroin to disguise the sweet taste of milk sugar, can be detected in the urine up to seventy-two hours after the last dose and provides circumstantial evidence of heroin use. Withdrawal from heroin for the addict consists of progression from yawning, tearing, dilated pupils in the early stages to restlessness, insomnia, generalized muscle cramps and "gooseflesh," and then to severe intestinal cramps, diarrhea, and sweating in the late stages. Occasionally, untreated withdrawal can progress to convulsions and, very rarely, to death from shock.

Because there was a recent report of a teen-ager who died of a heroin overdose while his parents thought he was just sleeping on the couch, it may be appropriate to describe these symptoms. The individual who has had an overdose is drowsy to unconscious, breathes at a slower rate than normal, may appear to have difficulty breathing, and may have a bluish hue around his lips. His pupils are very small and don't get smaller when a light is shined into them (try it on yourself to see the normal response). He doesn't need to have a needle mark, for overdose can happen from snorting (sniffing) heroin.

We have said that most teen-agers are poorly motivated to stop using heroin once they have begun. But what about those who are willing to try? The following are the current methods of treatment for heroin addicts:

METHADONE

Methadone is a synthetic opiate, similar in structure to heroin itself. Like heroin, it is addictive. Why, then, is it used?

It has an advantage over heroin in that it can be taken by mouth rather than by injection, is long-acting so that it only need be given once a day rather than the usual three times a day for heroin, does not cloud the mind or produce the "high" of heroin, and in sufficient dosage can even block the heroin high if the ex-addict tries to use it while taking methadone.

Withdrawal from methadone is also easier and less painful than that from heroin.

Methadone is currently being used in two distinct ways in the treatment of heroin addicts. The first is for detoxification. The addict is placed on a dose of methadone sufficient to satisfy his craving for heroin and to prevent the onset of withdrawal symptoms. The dose is then decreased gradually on a daily basis over a one- to two-week period, depending on the size of the heroin habit. At the end of this predetermined period the methadone is stopped completely and the patient experiences no physical signs of withdrawal. The "drug hunger" usually persists, however, and it is generally agreed that detoxification must be followed by supportive therapy and rehabilitation.

The controversy surrounding methadone pertains rather to its use for "maintenance." The theory behind methadone maintenance is that the addict is ill and requires medication for his illness. He is usually compared with the diabetic, who needs his daily insulin in order to function and, once having gotten it, is indistinguishable from a healthy individual. The addict is given a daily methadone dose at a hospital clinic and can then attend school or work without the former fear and activity related to obtaining heroin. There is no cost to the patient, and the actual cost for a dose of methadone is two cents compared to heroin habits, which can run as high as $100 a day.

The methadone maintenance program was developed at the Rockefeller University by Dr. Vincent Dole, a bio-chemist, and Dr. Marie Nyswander, a psychiatrist, and is now more than six years old. Roughly two-thirds of the close to four thousand patients now in the program have remained off heroin, and drug-related crimes, such as robbery, have been dramatically cut for those so treated.

Those who object to methadone maintenance claim that to use it is merely to substitute one addiction for another. Others feel that it treats the symptom, not the cause, and that with proper therapy the addict can be freed of all addiction.

Until recently a person would not be accepted for the program unless he was over twenty years of age and addicted for a minimum of three years. Now that more funds are becoming available for enlarging the program, the age limits are being relaxed. While few may object to placing a forty-five-year-old ex-con addict on methadone, it is quite a different situation when the person in question is a fifteen-year-old heroin user of three months. Of more concern to us, however, is the lack of experience with the physical effects of methadone on the adolescent. As indicated previously, heroin, similar in composition to methadone, has a more devastating effect on the endocrine system of the teen-ager than that of the adult, and it is quite possible that the same is true of methadone.

"SELF-HELP" OR GROUP THERAPY PROGRAMS

These are residential treatment programs that utilize ex-addicts and techniques of peer-pressure to help addicts to get off heroin and other drugs. The prototype of this approach is Synanon, which was established in 1958. Communities of addicts at various stages of the rehabilitation process use group confrontation to break down the defenses of the addict, tolerating none of the manipulative behavior so characteristic of the addict's relationship with professionals and those unfamiliar with the drug subculture. The ultimate goal is to rebuild his ego. After a usual period of eighteen months the successful ex-addict is ready to go out from the sheltered community environment to the temptations of life on "the street." Most of the graduates of such programs find employment in similar settings. Statistics for success rates are difficult to obtain, but most agree that more than half of those who enter leave within the first three months. Many teen-agers cannot tolerate the rigid structure of these programs, and often lacking insight, recoil under the sometimes brutal verbal methods used to expose their character defects in the presence of their peers.

Nonetheless, of those currently available, this type of approach seems one of the best suited to the peer-conscious adolescent. The regional field office of the National Institute of Mental Health listed in the Appendix can supply you with names of facilities utilizing these methods in your area.

INDIVIDUAL PSYCHOTHERAPY

It is generally agreed that this form of therapy is only suited to the heroin user with an underlying psychiatric problem. Teen-agers usually don't respond optimally to individual therapy, but rather to the group approach. There are, however, some therapists with unique talent who do extremely well with teen-agers with drug-related problems. Your local county medical society or medical-school department of adolescent psychiatry can provide you with names of psychiatrists who specialize in teen-agers.

CONSULTATIVE SERVICES

These provide a comprehensive approach to the factors responsible for drug abuse in any one individual. Psychological testing, aptitude testing, psychiatric evaluation, vocational guidance, and remedial reading may be offered in such a program. The emphasis of this therapy is usually not drugs per se, but the correction of causative factors. The in-depth nature of these programs creates long waiting lists. In addition, most are privately run, so cost may be another deterrent.

INVOLUNTARY DETENTION

All facilities thus far discussed are voluntary in nature. The teen-ager must be motivated in order to enroll, and it is obvious that the degree of success depends on the extent of the motivation. The most difficult problems arise, however, with the adolescents who are unable to undertake a program of change.

For the sake of completeness, we should mention that facilities now exist in New York State and elsewhere for the involuntary detention of heroin users, apart from facilities for other offenders. This last resort is usually left for the teen-ager who has tried various programs and dropped out and who is involved in criminal activity to support his habit. Commitment can be initiated by family, citizens, or those within the court system.

It is an old adage in medicine that when many therapies exist for any one ailment, it means that none works, for if it did only one would be necessary. Perhaps it is too early to know which one that is in the area of therapy for drug abuse, but all will agree that the best approach is prevention. There is much that parents and teen-agers themselves can do in the area of prevention. This is vividly demonstrated in the program created by a town in Westchester County, New York, under the direction of one of our colleagues.

Here is how the community went about it:

1. Anonymous questionnaires were distributed by students to assess the extent and types of drugs used.
2. Community meetings were held with consultants available for questions and answers, as well as small seminars for parents and teen-agers on various aspects of drug abuse.
3. The school library was set up with current source material relevant to various drugs and toxins. These were chosen by consultants to present all information on controversial topics, not just that covering harmful effects.
4. A course on drugs was taught by the school psychologist, nurse, science teacher, and health education teacher.
5. Those teen-agers who were found to be heavily involved in addictive drugs formed the core of a separate program. They were seen individually

and together with their parents by the school guidance counselor, and a program of ongoing therapy was initiated. When the school records of these boys and girls were reviewed, it was apparent that they had performed poorly in comparison with their siblings for many years before drug use began. Remedial reading and tutoring were given to those found in need.

6. There were evening "bull-sessions," for those teen-agers on drugs led by practicing psychiatrists in the community.

7. A "hot-line"—a telephone service manned by doctors, lawyers, pharmacists, clergy, and other interested citizens—was initiated in the evening hours. Although this was originally set up for teen-agers with "bad trips" or drug overdoses, they began to call anonymously with problems ranging from fear of pregnancy to worry over parental marital problems. When the nature of the call was such as to require more than just "someone to talk to," the callers were referred to competent professionals in that or neighboring communities for specific services. Police officials cooperated with the program.

8. There was a system of monitoring and re-evaluation: questionnaires were recirculated every six months to identify new problem areas and to check progress in those previously identified.

9. A "narcotics council" made up of clergymen, doctors, and lawyers, was set up to advise and supervise activities.

One school system in California set up a program in which the focus was the school ombudsman. He was a teacher with no special background in drug-abuse problems, but was chosen because he was the one to whom the students turned spontaneously when they had difficulties. He was freed of all classroom activity and given training that ranged from working on a crew responsible for burning marijuana fields to visiting the morgue with pathologists studying drug-overdose deaths to sitting in at group therapy sessions at one of the self-help programs.

All agree that the key to a successful prevention program is education and involvement of the kids themselves from the inception of the program. Indeed, the students at one Eastern Ivy League college, alarmed at the death of a girl from sniffing heroin, started what is considered a very successful campaign to rid the campus of heroin. No adults were involved at all.

The Hallucinogens

"In an aggressive society potent hallucinogens are likely to enhance belligerence; in a peaceful society the same drugs can be expected to produce passivity and introspection." With this statement Dr. Donald Louria, an articulate observer of the drug scene, emphasizes the importance of cultural and social influences on the effects of psychedelic drugs. To generalize about this growing group of substances would be to oversimplify. Instead we will list each such "drug" and indicate what is known about it at this time. Some, such as the mushrooms of Mexico, have been known to man for their psychedelic powers for centuries. Others, like LSD, are man-made and a product of the technology of the twentieth century.

NATURALLY OCCURRING HALLUCINOGENS

Marijuana

This, the most commonly used hallucinogen, was dealt with earlier.

Peyote (Mescaline)

This substance, which appears to be supplanting LSD in popularity, is derived from a cactus plant found in Texas and Mexico. The heads of the plant are removed and dried and then chewed or brewed into tea.

First used in pre-Columbian times, it became the

basis for the founding in 1885 of the Native American Church by more than fifty Indian tribes.

Although taken for the visual, olfactory, and auditory hallucinations and trancelike states it produces, all its effects are not pleasant. Immediately after ingesting the dried button, the user experiences nausea. This is followed by drying of the lips and tongue, drying and flushing of the skin, inability to focus the eyes due to dilation of the pupils, insomnia, and restlessness. Numbness, chest pains, headache, and uterine contractions similar to menstrual cramps may occur. In serious cases severe diarrhea, copious nasal discharge, and an unpleasant body odor are noted. As with all hallucinogens, the psychic experiences may occasionally be terrifying ones, and a manic-depressive psychosis after use of peyote has been reported. The usual duration of action of this agent is six to twelve hours, but some observers claim that its effects may last for days. It is not considered to be an addictive drug.

Mescal Beans

Mescal beans are no longer popular among the Indians who originally espoused them for their hallucinogenic and medicinal properties, presumably because of the convulsions and occasional death from respiratory failure they also caused. The beans are the seeds of a shrub *(Sophora secundiflora)* found in the same areas as are peyote plants. They are mentioned here only because of the similarity between their name and mescaline, which is used popularly.

Nutmeg

The seed of the apricot-like fruit of the tropical tree *Myristica fragrans,* nutmeg has long been known for its hallucinogenic properties. In the usual dose of one teaspoon, visual hallucinations may occur. More characteristic, however, is its ability to produce a feeling of detachment and distortion of time and space perception. Because the dose necessary to produce the

desired effects is close to that which causes dryness of
the mouth, headache, rapid pulse, nausea, dizziness,
and shortness of breath, nutmeg is usually considered
a "last resort" to be ingested only when marijuana is
not available. Its effects last for a day or two.

Morning Glory Seeds

There are three species of morning glory plants
found in Mexico and the United States that produce
seeds with hallucinogenic properties. The seeds (usually fifteen per dose) are soaked in water before being
chewed. They have been found to contain a lysergic
acid derivative, thought to be one-twentieth as strong
as LSD. The effects are less constant than LSD, however, and some people never experience hallucinations
with their use.

Jimsonweed (Stramonium)

A mixture of the leaves, branches, and flowers of
this Western American plant has been used in the
treatment of asthma. Its ability to produce hallucinations is overshadowed by the effects of its major ingredient, atropine, which causes dryness of the mouth.
Similar to nutmeg, its popularity is limited by the
same unpleasant factors mentioned above.

Sacred Mushroom (Teonanacatl)

The active ingredient in this plant, known since an-
tiquity to produce hallucinations when chewed, now
appears to be psilocybin. Psilocybin is approximately
one-two-hundredth the strength of LSD and produces
similar effects according to a 1963 report in the jour-
nal *Psychiatry*.

SYNTHETIC HALLUCINOGENS

STP (2,5,-Dimethoxy-4-Methyl-Amphetamine)

According to Louria STP stands for Serenity, Tranquility, and Peace. Also known as DOM, this substance is taken orally and causes visual hallucinations

and psychosis similar to those produced by LSD, but lasting four to seven days. It is thus more powerful than LSD. Death from respiratory paralysis has been reported following use of STP. It is now apparent that much of the "street" STP is contaminated with atropine, which is probably responsible for this complication. The presence of atropine also presents another serious problem. "Bad trips" caused by the hallucinogens are usually treated with the tranquilizer Thorazine. The inadvertent combination of Thorazine and atropine has been responsible for the death of three patients so treated. The illicit drug user continuously risks consuming something other than what he thinks he has purchased.

DET (Di-ethyltryptamine)

A substance whose hallucinatory effect lasts two to three hours after smoking or injection.

DMT (Di-methyltryptamine)

A short-acting substance that produces hallucinations for less than one hour after smoking or injection.

THC (Tetrahydrocannabinol)

The synthesis of this compound followed its isolation as the active hallucinogenic principle in marijuana. Its effects are those of marijuana, but a tablet is five times as potent as a joint.

FUK

According to Drs. Lionel Solursh and Wilfrid Clement, this substance arrived on the streets of Canada in 1968. A phosgene derivative, its initials appear to have been more socially than chemically determined. Its effects are reportedly similar to those of LSD, but of slightly longer duration. It is available in capsule form. Little is yet known about possible adverse effects.

LSD (d-lysergic acid diethylamide-25)

From ergot, a fungus that grows on rye plants and is used medicinally to stop bleeding and migraine headaches, LSD was derived and synthesized in 1938. In his informative book *The Drug Scene* Dr. Donald Louria describes how Dr. Albert Hofmann discovered the hallucinogenic properties of this drug five years later by accidentally ingesting or inhaling it:

> "I felt strangely restless and dizzy. I lay down and sank into a not unpleasant delirium which was marked by an extreme degree of fantasy. In a sort of trance with closed eyes, fantastic visions of extraordinary vividness accompanied by a kaleidoscopic play of intense coloration continuously swirled around me."

In the years following Hofmann's discovery, much has been learned about this substance. A tablespoon of the colorless, odorless, and tasteless compound is sufficient to "turn on" three hundred thousand people to its hallucinogenic properties. From a tiny speck on a sugar cube, cookie, stamp, or blotter one can experience a melange of sensory phenomena that range from the magnificent to the bizarre, all of them reportedly overwhelming.

All the LSD ingested is excreted within ninety minutes, yet its immediate hallucinogenic effects persist for eight to twelve hours, and users have reported reliving entire "trips" as long as a year later. These observations indicate that the drug acts by an indirect alteration of brain cells, caused by changes in serotonin, a chemical within these cells. While not addictive, LSD use is dangerous for other reasons. Its psychological effects are such that some people panic during a "bad trip" or a recurrence of one and may, if so predisposed, become psychotic. The unreality attendant on a trip has occasionally been responsible for the users falling great distances, thinking that they could fly. LSD has been shown in laboratory experiments to cause breakage of chromosomes, therefore it is potentially capable of producing birth defects. The fact that few individuals use this substance without also using other drugs makes reports of actual birth defects difficult to interpret. Claims by LSD cultists of the drug's aphrodisiac properties are disproved by Louria, who presents convincing evidence that actual sexual experiences under its influence are far from satisfactory. The possibility of chromosomal defects from LSD appears to be the rationale for many college students forsaking the drug in favor of mescaline, now the more popular hallucinogen. It has been our experience that LSD is also not popular with ghetto teenagers. One possible explanation for this may be that they prefer heroin, which allows them to escape from their bleak reality, to LSD, which is allegedly taken to assist in exploring reality. The simplest explanation is probably one of relative availability of each substance.

If someone is using LSD or mescaline, or sniffing glue or cleaning fluid, he will appear detached and unnaturally cheerful, and/or fearful, and will answer questions inappropriately. Then again, many parents think their teen-agers are doing that most of the time anyway. Unless they are under the influence of the toxin while being examined, it is difficult to prove its use. At the present time there is no reliable urine or blood test for detection of these substances.

Amphetamines

The tranquility, peace, and brotherhood of love once so unique to the Haight-Ashbury section of San Francisco is gone. In its place fear and paranoia run rampant, and the roar of the motorcycle gangs fills the air. What has transpired to effect this metamorphosis in less than two short years? The change is a chemical one. It is a change from the world of pot and LSD to that of speed.

"Speed" is the term given to methamphetamine or methedrine, a stimulant, when it is injected into the veins. It is the same substance that, as benzedrine, dexedrine, or preludin, may be sitting in your medicine cabinet at this moment. You may have used it to curb your appetite when dieting, or you may be taking between ten and fifteen mgs a day as a mood elevator. If you were in college in the late forties or early fifties, you may have used it to help you cram for an exam. Amphetamines must be dispensed by prescription, but it is apparent that they are easily available to those with the money to pay for them.

If taken occasionally by mouth, amphetamines make you more energetic, help you think clearly and sharply, make you more articulate, and reduce your desire for food. If they are taken by mouth on a daily basis, these effects tend to wear off, and the user needs more and more to produce the desired effect. With these larger doses, mood changes are often experienced, and frightening hallucinations frequently follow. These phenomena are exaggerated when amphetamines are injected into a vein, but it is by this route that an immediate, dramatic effect is experienced.

Initially there is a generalized full-body shock, compared by many users to a total orgasm. This is followed by racing of the pulse, heightening of the blood pressure, blurring of vision, and dilation of the pupils of the eyes. Activity is increased, sleep is impossible, and appetite is lost, as is the ability to concentrate. While on a speed binge, the user often becomes suspicious, and paranoid thoughts frequently develop. When coming down from a speed binge, or "crashing," he experiences a profound fatigue and depression. If more is unobtainable, a long period of sleep, often for two to three days, follows. Often during this period paranoid thoughts are exaggerated. The user often imagines that someone is out to kill him, and may decide to kill before he is killed. During a crash he is unable to do anything about these thoughts, but upon recovery, he may have the energy to do so. It is out of this phenomenon rather than the effect of the drug on the user per se that the admonition "speed kills" has arisen.

Amphetamines are not technically addictive in that they do not produce a typical picture of withdrawal when they are stopped. Brain-wave tests do, however, demonstrate changes associated with discontinuance of amphetamines in chronic users. That those changes are reversed when the drug is reintroduced suggests a form of addiction.

A teen-ager using amphetamines or "ups" appears to have boundless energy, unless he is "coming down," in which case he will sleep continuously for days. One on amphetamines has dilated pupils, a rapid pulse and respiratory rate, and an elevated blood pressure. He talks rapidly, with animation, but frequently makes no sense. Amphetamines can be detected in the urine by appropriate laboratory tests.

Psychological complications are not the only detrimental effects of amphetamine abuse. Hepatitis resulting from the use of an unsterilized needle is just as much a danger to the speed shooter as to the heroin user. Brain hemorrhages are seen in those who die from overdoses of this drug. Recent reports of neurologic impairment in young adult abusers suggests that the high-blood-pressure effects may also take their toll gradually in those who inject amphetamines intravenously.

The number of amphetamine abusers is unknown. A study of medical students at a western school by Smith and Blechly in 1965 indicated that almost half had tried amphetamines more than once. In 1968 it was reported that 22 percent of the upper graders in a San Francisco high school had experimented with the drug. A year later in Toronto a study revealed that more than 7 percent of students between the seventh and thirteenth grades of high school had recently used stimulants. It would appear then that amphetamine use is second only to marijuana, according to these studies. It has been our own experience that amphetamine abuse is quite rare in the New York inner-city-ghetto teen-age population, but more common in the suburban areas of the city.

Cocaine

Among archaeological discoveries in Peru have been artifacts showing faces with bulging cheeks. These are believed to portray the Incas' practice of chewing the leaf of the coca plant. The "abuse" of cocaine, as it is now known, is not new. What is, and what makes this practice more dangerous now than in the past, is the amount and route of administration of this drug. Whereas the ancient custom was to chew the leaf of the plant, resulting in marked local, but minimal, concentration in the blood-stream, it is now usually injected. In order to sustain its exhilarating effects, cocaine is frequently injected repeatedly within an hour's time. Because it diminishes hunger, the chronic user may be malnourished. He is in danger of undertaking tasks beyond his physical capabilities because of an imagined increase in strength while on the drug. Infections can result at the site of injection, little attention being paid to sterilization technique. As with amphetamines, to which it is functionally similar, the abuser may develop paranoid delusions. Rarer complications include convulsions and death from respiratory paralysis.

What appears to have saved teen-agers from the pattern of repetitive administration seen in adults seems to be the cost. Cocaine reportedly sells for fifty dollars a gram (about five capsules of crystalline powder). The more popular use of cocaine in the teen-agers we treat is in conjunction with heroin. A capsule of cocaine is injected intravenously with each dose of heroin, usually three times a day, the combination being called a "speedball." Cocaine is not physically addictive, but the desire for its effects renders the user psychologically addicted.

Barbiturates

This group of compounds act on the central nervous system to depress all bodily functions. As a result, one who uses barbiturates becomes drowsy, and his pulse rate, blood pressure, and rate of breathing are lowered. If you think of the effects of amphetamines and appreciate that those of barbiturates are the exact opposite, you will understand why the former are referred to as "ups" and the latter "downs."

Barbiturates are used medically as tranquilizers, pain killers, anti-hypertensives, and most often as convulsion-preventives for epileptics. It is this last property that has important implications for a barbiturate abuser; for if he should stop taking them without medical supervision, he is likely to suffer a convulsion with resultant brain damage or death. For this reason withdrawal from barbiturates is the most dangerous of all drugs and requires gradual detoxification in a hospital setting. The other significant danger of barbiturate abuse is that of an overdose, which is usually fatal.

It has always been an engima that teen-agers would desire a substance that would depress rather than exhilarate. In fact, until very recently "downs" were usually used solely in conjunction with heroin because they allegedly sustained its effect, or to help one "come down" from an amphetamine high. It was not until early 1970 that we began to see adolescents addicted to barbiturates alone. Most of our patients started using barbiturates as self-medication for insomnia which resulted from mass-media variety anxiety or that caused by withdrawal from other drugs, particularly heroin. They are usually administered by the oral route in doses upward of 50 mg. Commonly abused are the shorter-acting barbiturates such as seconal, nembutal, and amytal.

All that has been described for the barbiturates applies equally to other sleeping pills, the most popular of which is CIBA (Doriden).

A youngster taking barbiturates or "downs" may have small pupils, slow pulse, and low blood pressure, and he will appear depressed. Barbiturates can also be detected in the urine by appropriate laboratory tests.

DEPRESSION

No one in the course of his life escapes completely some period of depression, and perhaps no group is more vulnerable to it than the adolescent group. There are features of depression common to all ages from childhood to old age, but their outward manifestations may be somewhat different in the adolescent. It is the particular vulnerability combined with a misleading outward appearance that makes depression in the adolescent both important and yet difficult to recognize.

Depression is, in the first place, the most painful of all psychic experiences. The victim, and we use that word advisedly, experiences a sense of despair, not merely sadness, a deep, black gloom, as if he is trapped. He has feelings not only of hopelessness, but of helplessness. He is sad because he has lost something—love, self-esteem, a job, a body organ, a limb—or his loss may be imaginary. He may feel that someone does not love him or that people do not think highly of him. The important point to remember is how the victim of this disability feels, not the realities of the situation, if you are to empathize with him.

Accompanying this sense of loss is a sense of rage. The sufferer is angry about his loss. In dealing with a depressed teen-ager, it is important to be aware of this element of anger. It is one of the things we sense, and it is one of the feelings we perceive coming from the depressed person that turns us off.

Take this sense of loss, then add on to it rage, and blend it with a sense of unworthiness. Imagine then that the rage is turned against the person himself. He blames himself for the loss; he was not worthy of the love he lost. And this adds up to the unbearable feeling of despair we call depression.

At the time that he is feeling the depression, the sufferer can see "no way out." His time sense is disordered because he can see no future. If he could envisage other possibilities in the future, he would not be depressed. "This too shall pass" is not in the vocabulary of the teen-ager in despair.

In general it is quite likely, though not inevitable, that a young person will in conversation give hints of this psychic dilemma, if he does not identify it outright.

"I feel down" or "I am in the dumps" are kind of psychic geographical locations of a feeling whose sense of lowness is conveyed by the word depression. It is the opposite of "I am up in the clouds" or "I am high."

The depressed teen-ager will also express feelings of unworthiness: "I am no good"; "I deserve it"; "I feel like a piece of dirt." These are all manifestations of low self-esteem.

An obvious slowing-down movement is common in depressed adults. In the presence of good health, an individual will appear tired and listless. He may after a fair night's sleep feel extremely tired in the morning but pick up as the day goes on. Although this is usually the case with the depressed adolescent, he may not feel better as the day goes on and may spend a sleepness night.

In addition, and more striking, is the fact that the depressed young person may not be slowed down in his activities but indeed be more active. He may pace nervously or run around ineffectively from activity to activity.

There are times when a person with depression is occupied sufficiently or even preoccupied with school or political activities so that he will show very little evidence of his low state. But when these activities are not available to him, he will show the more typical signs of depression. This accounts for holiday blues and for the fact, for example, that more suicides occur during holidays or on Sundays. We shall be discussing suicides later.

The depressed person may appear obviously sad, eyes lowered, mouth turned down, moving slowly, speaking in muted tones. He may wear a mask. He may smile, but it is not a genuine smile. Most people can spot it. Lips are pulled in a straight, taut line across the teeth, giving a mechanical, tight appearance in contrast to the more flowing, curving appearance of the natural smile. His voice may appear forced and unnaturally cheerful. There is something unauthentic about the whole image. It used to be said of depressed people that they were unkempt. This sign is no longer useful, for surely if we relied on it we would overdiagnose depression.

If one is depressed and can identify it, he should try to be objective. It is important in the first instance to know that a feeling of depression, whatever its cause, is temporary. It may last a week or a year, but it will pass. In saying whatever its cause, we meant to indicate that a feeling of depression could have a physical cause (see Chapter 8). In addition, a feeling of depression is a common aftereffect of various drugs: barbiturates, alcohol, amphetamines.

Therefore, the first thing to do is to see a doctor, even—and most probably—if the adolescent has to be dragged there. At the very least, he can rule out a physical disorder.

Let us assume that there is no physical cause. Then what?

The first thing to know on a reasoning level, even if it cannot be known on an emotional level, is that a depression is a symptom which is *temporary*. Despite the fact that the victim cannot see an end to it, particularly in the young person it is likely to leave in relatively short order. Depression by our definition includes the fact that the sufferer does not *feel* this. Indeed, if he did, he would not feel depressed.

It is difficult for most of us both to bear depression ourselves and to bear witness to it. We are angry at ourselves as if we are depressed, and we sense it in the depressed one. It is important to be aware of this.

When someone says to a depressed person, "Buck up, what do you have to be depressed about?" not only is this sure to be useless, but even more, in reflecting our own impatience and resentment, it is sure to be damaging. It is often better to be silently compassionate than to try to be "helpful."

Insight therapy, sorting out the dynamic factors that have produced the despair, may be needed if there is not some spontaneous resolution. A seriously depressed person should be in the hands of a skilled psychotherapist.

It is not uncommon for physicians to use drugs in depression, since depression can lead to suicide. The drugs commonly used, imipramine and nortryptyline, while effective in elevating the mood of a depressed person, are not hallucinogens, do not cause pleasurable sensations, nor do they cause a high.

To sum up, depression is a temporary state that occurs when someone experiences a sense of loss—usually for the teen-ager it is a feeling of loss of love—for which he blames himself. This gloom, accompanied by anger directed at himself, results in psychic pain or depression. It is important, indeed crucial, for the depressed person and his friends and family to see this as temporary and commonplace. Furthermore, it can always be helped.

SUICIDE

The juxtaposition of these sections on depression and suicide represents a logical sequence. That too little attention has been paid to this fact is tragically apparent in the fact that suicide is one of the leading causes of death among adolescents. If one were to include at least some of the deaths from automobile accidents as suicide, perhaps unconsciously masked as accident-proneness, the figures would be even more awesome.

Regardless of how one measures the death toll, it is extremely important to recognize the potential suicide in order to prevent it. This is even more urgent with adolescents, because in this group suicide is more often impulsive and less likely to be a reflection of a more or less permanent decision, such as one made by someone who is chronically ill.

It is true that there are one hundred more attempts than there are suicides; but one out of one hundred represents a real possibility, and there is no way of predicting which young person who speaks of ending his life will actually do so.

There are differences in motivation and method between boys and girls. Girls are likely to attempt suicide in situations in which they feel that they may be abandoned by a loved figure. A history of previous hurtful separations—from a father, for example—is likely to sensitize them so that a later threat, whether real or imaginary, of abandonment by a boyfriend may be the cause of a suicide attempt. Stated another way, the threat of loss of love from a significant other person may motivate a girl to commit suicide.

A girl, usually conceiving of herself in our culture as passive and in need of the love of others, is in some contradistinction to a boy, whose self-esteem is threatened by some real or imaginary limitation of his capacity to take care of himself. Such a threat to his potency or his ability to care for himself may be the event that leads him to self-destruction.

Although girls may make more attempts, boys are more often successful—if that is the correct word. In addition boys are more likely to use violent means such as guns and hanging, whereas girls are more likely to use pills.

It is important to be able to recognize the potential suicide in yourself or in others. Every suicide attempt is a cry for help. The idea is to help before the attempt.

Anyone who talks of suicide should be taken seriously, particularly if there is a history of a previous suicide gesture or a history of accident-proneness. Adolescents are particularly suggestible. Given a vulnerably depressed teen-ager who reads or hears of some dramatic news featuring suicide, the likelihood of an attempt is increased. More suicide attempts are made on holidays and weekends than at other times, perhaps because the absence of normal routine makes the individual more aware of his loneliness.

Any expression of hopelessness, helplessness, and despair should be regarded with suspicion.

The tendency of a person to isolate himself or to be isolated often precedes the suicide attempt.

A period of calm, perhaps resignation, that follows in the wake of a depression may indicate a decision to commit suicide, and hence should not lull one into a false sense of security.

It is of utmost importance to refrain from remarks such as "You have everything to live for" or exhortations such as "Pull yourself together." They are only likely to be destructive and may even be misinterpreted as a challenge to carry out the act.

Indeed, and we hesitate to mention this for fear of offending some, we must all look into our own souls when we are faced with a potential suicide and examine our own true attitudes toward him. If you come up with some sense of hostility to someone making the threat, it is best to be honest and not try to "help" him in this way. You are more likely to harm, whatever your conscious intention. The thought of such a possibility is shocking, but nevertheless there is some psychiatric evidence, tenuous though it is, that this is indeed often the case. It does appear that prolonged contact with someone who is depressed and who threatens suicide can result in a "Well, let him get it over with" attitude.

If immediate psychiatric care is not readily available, as is frequently the case, one may turn to the suicide-prevention centers that now exist in many cities. Numbers to call are listed in the Appendix. Many hospitals have walk-in emergency psychiatric consultation. A physician should also be consulted.

The person with the suspected suicidal intent

should not be left alone. He should also be spoken to directly about his intentions. There used to be a prevalent idea that speaking about suicide to someone contemplating it might precipitate it. This is not true. It is best to confront the person and ask directly whether it is on his mind. He may indeed be helped by this.

Remember, suicide attempts are pleas for help. Failure to recognize this and act accordingly is indeed tragic.

CHAPTER ELEVEN

The Psychology of Adolescence

A CATECHISM FOR ADOLESCENCE

Why is there so much trouble with adolescents today?

The best way to understand the turbulence of contemporary adolescence is to see it as three simultaneous revolutions: a biological one, a psychological one, and a sociological one.

What is the biological revolution?

The biological revolution starts when areas in the brain no longer keep certain hormone-secreting glands in check. Prior to adolescence there are some little-understood areas in the brain and a structure called the pineal gland that inhibit the sex glands. We know this to be true because certain kinds of brain damage, or a tumor that destroys the pineal gland, will unleash the glands, resulting in sexual precocity. This can occur in very early childhood.

Once the inhibitory forces are weakened, a series of events takes place resulting in very rapid biological changes with subsequent obvious psychological changes.

What specifically happens is that an area at the base of the brain, the hypothalamus, apparently sends nerve impulses, or messages, to the master gland, the pituitary, which in turn releases its own hormone, a growth hormone, and directs or stimulates the sex glands: the ovary in the female, the testes in the male, and the adrenal glands in both sexes.

Structurally, in general, rapid growth follows, with development of the sex organs and secondary sexual characteristics. We have detailed this in Chapter One.

There are direct consequences of this in terms of behavior in the form of an increase in physical restlessness (usually in the form of aggressiveness), increased sexual activity, short attention span, and the development of the capacity for abstract thinking.

Can biological changes change the way we think?

The Swiss psychologist Piaget believes that thinking in general develops out of an organic matrix. Specifically, the organizational changes that result from adolescence make possible abstract thinking. This provides a biological explanation for the almost ubiquitous concern of adolescence with idealism, religion, justice, or chess for that matter.

Is the biological revolution any different now than it was a hundred years ago?

There is some evidence that adolescence is occurring somewhat earlier now than it did a century ago. This is due, of course, in great part to better nutrition. This would also explain why adolescents today are bigger and stronger. The biological revolution is more overwhelming now than perhaps it has ever been.

What about the psychological revolution?

The psychological revolution always follows the biological revolution. Before we try to understand this revolution, let us agree on how we want to describe it. It is particularly difficult to describe a mental or internal experience. We must always use some kind of metaphor. This is clear when we remember that we commonly use in relationship to internal or mental experiences such terms as "I am upset," "He had a breakdown," or more contemporaneously, "He is a square," "She is groovy," or "They are uptight." Because our vision of the world is changing, we are perhaps more prone to use spatial metaphors to describe mental events or concepts than we were in the past.

To exist literally means to stand out, to occupy a position in space. Even to express the very fact of our being we use a spatial metaphor.

We all exist; that is, we have a position. Adolescence represents a marked change in position, second only to birth in its magnitude. In fact, being adolescent is almost like being reborn, and many adolescents think of it that way.

The adolescent does not necessarily want to change position; he must. As we stated, the biological revolution precedes the psychological one. The bodily changes, the increase in size, the increase in glandular activity, all create new instincts that must be gratified. The adolescent perceives these new instincts as sensations or feelings that are vague and diffuse and cause him to be restless.

Before adolescence we do exist in a kind of fantasy. We see ourselves as children, usually in relationship to our parents. We are in a position of being children, which means we usually have someone who will support us, someone we are tied to. The new fantasies of adolescence change our view of what we want our position to be. We, of course, do not use the term fantasy in a "sick" sense, but rather to describe our mental image of ourselves in relationship to other people. Fantasies only become "sick" when they are far removed from reality. As our fantasy lives in response to instinctual needs brought on by changing biological conditions, we develop a new construction of ourselves. It is in this reconstruction during adolescence that our position as a child becomes untenable—yet we have not found for ourselves a new position.

The adolescent is in a sort of limbo. He is neither a child nor an adult. He has no fixed position. This accounts for his sensitivity. Any disturbance, even seemingly slight, is bound to upset him or to move him.

Why do adolescents always seem to be ashamed?

Traditionally we have assumed that their sense of shame was due to guilt, and more specifically guilt over masturbation, but this is probably not so. What we think is going on, putting ourselves in their position, is that the sense of shame is really a fear of being exposed.

Many adolescents seem to want to withdraw. Some feel particularly ashamed when they are with their parents in public. They feel that not only they but their parents also are exposed for all their peers to see and presumably to scorn. That is why they are so self-conscious.

They are literally aware of their new selves, and they must feel terribly vulnerable.

If we accept that in their new position they are more susceptible to non-existence, to non-being—if we understand furthermore that man conceives of non-being not only as biological death but also as spiritual non-existence, as feeling meaningless, and moral non-existence, as being condemned by his fellow man—we can understand some of the adolescent preoccupation.

The adolescent handles the problem of biological non-being, real death, with bravado. Many have a feeling of omnipotence, which if they act it out takes the form of risk-taking and perhaps drug usage. They are not physically afraid.

Spiritually they are markedly preoccupied with the meaning of life, or rather the contemporary meaninglessness of life. Their concern with spirituality ranges from militant atheism to Hinduism, sometimes unfortunately aided by drugs.

They are confused sometimes to a point at which it is difficult to tell whether a great deal of their mental experiences and consequent behavior is normal development or represents mental illness. As Anna Freud has stated, "Adolescence is by its nature an interruption of peaceful growth, and the upholding of a steady equilibrium during this process is in itself abnormal.

"The adolescent manifestations come close to symptom formation of the neurotic, psychotic, or dissocial order and merge almost imperceptibly into borderline states, initial frustrate or full-fledged forms of all the mental illnesses. Consequently the differential diagnosis between the adolescent upsets and true pathology becomes a difficult task.

". . . in the majority of cases, the manifestations of the adolescent process are not predictable since they depend almost wholly on quantitative relation, *i.e.* on the suddenness of drive increase, the corresponding increase in anxiety causing all the rest of the upheaval."

It is plain that many events have occurred to upset the adolescent, and it is sometimes difficult even for experts to tell whether he is mentally ill or merely experiencing and behaving in a way that means he is finding a new position. We suppose that is what is meant by his or her bad or good disposition.

What is the position of the parents in all of this?

Parents do not have it easy either. They have their own needs in relation to the child. Perhaps this quote from Rabbi Kabia, who lived in ancient times, will help us see this more clearly: "My son, more than a calf wishes to suck does the cow yearn to suckle." In childhood there are reciprocal needs between parent and child, the former to give support, the latter to lean. All of this gets upset at adolescence.

This seems to explain in large part the ambivalently strained relationship between teen-agers and parents. On the one hand the parent needs to have the child dependent, at the same time knowing that he must at some point let go. On the other hand, in complementary fashion, the adolescent needs support yet fears engulfment ("You people are smothering me") in his struggle to establish his new independent revolution.

What about the sociological revolution?

The sociological revolution explains in large part why adolescence today is different than it was a hundred years ago. The biological revolution and the psychological revolution have always been with us, but society has in the final analysis determined their courses. In general, societies can be said to go through inhibitory and remissive phases. Inhibitory societies act in conflict with the individual. A remissive society, such as ours today, grants more freedom of action.

In past societies there were always prohibitions against sexual gratification, particularly for women. Sex was not supposed to be enjoyable for them; it was for the purpose of begetting children. Sex for fun was, if practiced covertly, overtly frowned upon. Our society is no longer, in general, prohibitive about sex—any form of it. This change in attitude has followed certain medical advances—particularly The Pill, which has made sex for pleasure possible—but the effect is the same. Society no longer inhibits the individual. There are other examples.

In the past most of us saw our lives in a linear fashion—we had to "keep in line." We assumed that there was a course, or path, that we were expected to take. This path was different for each socio-economic group.

Saying it in another way, we were supposed to follow in our parents' footsteps. Now all of that has been knocked over. The path is no longer straight ahead and upward. For many there are no gratifications to be deferred until they "reach the top." Rather, they see themselves as out in the flat. Each day is a thing unto itself. Whereas in the past society's needs superseded those of the individual, many today look at society, the establishment, as the outright enemy of the individual. This is a relatively new phenomenon. In a sense, whether right or wrong, the purpose of life has shifted from service to society to self-service.

It should be clear how this new social situation makes it easier for the adolescent to act out his fantasies and how it makes it harder for the parent, unaided by a consensus society, to hold him in check. When the older generation states, "We always listened to our parents," we must remember that it was not the voice of the parent alone that was heard, but the voice of the whole society in harmony.

What is the answer to the strains between adolescents and parents today?

There is, unfortunately, a prevalent and quite destructive fantasy in our society—namely, that there *is* an answer. Indeed, the unfulfilled quest for the "answer" is the cause of suffering. Far more useful would be a quest for understanding.

It has been said of contemporary adolescents that they alone are at home in the world. Born into a technological age, the age of rapid communications, space exploration, computers, and medical advances, all of which change and promise so much, they are at the same time the indigenous, the parents, and the strangers.

That is only, however, part of it. Remember, they are born into a new world without a sense of tradition or continuity, with no road maps to guide them; they are the forlorns of this world. It has been said of contemporary man that he must invent his future. He must find the new balance between the desires of the individual, the needs of the family, and the needs of society.

APPENDICES

A Guide To Medical Clinics
For Adolescents

THE UNITED STATES OF AMERICA

ALABAMA

Adolescent Unit
University of Alabama Medical Center
Birmingham, Alabama

CALIFORNIA

Division of Adolescent Medicine
Children's Hospital of Los Angeles
4650 Sunset Boulevard
Los Angeles, California

Adolescent Clinic
Kaiser Foundation Hospital
Los Angeles, California

Adolescent Service
Children's Hospital
2820-15th Avenue
San Francisco, California

Youth Clinic
Children's Hospital of San Francisco
3641 California Street
San Francisco, California

Youth Clinic
Presbyterian Medical Center
2340 Clay Street
San Francisco, California

COLORADO

Adolescent Clinic
University of Colorado Medical Center
4200 East Ninth Avenue
Denver, Colorado

Youth Center
Children's Hospital
370 Ash Street
Denver, Colorado

CONNECTICUT

Medical Program for Adolescents
Yale University School of Medicine
333 Cedar Street
New Haven, Connecticut

DISTRICT OF COLUMBIA

Adolescent Clinic
Children's Hospital of D.C.
2125-13th Street, N.W.
Washington, D.C.

Adolescent Medicine Service
Walter Reed General Hospital
Washington, D.C.

GEORGIA

Medical College of Georgia
Augusta, Georgia

HAWAII

Straub Clinic
888 South King Street
Honolulu, Hawaii

Kauikeolani Children's Hospital
226 N. Kaukini Street
Honolulu, Hawaii

ILLINOIS

Adolescent Clinic
Loyola University Hospital
Maywood, Illinois

KENTUCKY

Department of Pediatrics
University of Kentucky
Lexington, Kentucky

MARYLAND

Adolescent Service
Johns Hopkins Hospital
Baltimore, Maryland

Adolescent Clinic
University of Maryland Hospital
Baltimore, Maryland

MASSACHUSETTS

The Adolescents' Unit
Children's Hospital Medical Center
300 Longwood Avenue
Boston, Massachusetts

Adolescent Medicine Seminar
Kennedy Memorial Hospital
30 Warren Street
Brighton, Massachusetts

Mount Auburn Hospital
330 Mt. Aubern Street
Cambridge, Massachusetts

MICHIGAN

Adolescent Clinic
University Hospital
Ann Arbor, Michigan

MINNESOTA

Teenage Medical Clinic
2425 Chicago Avenue, S.
Minneapolis, Minnesota

NEBRASKA

Adolescent Unit
University of Nebraska College of Medicine Hospital
Lincoln, Nebraska

Adolescent Clinic
Children's Memorial Hospital
3925 Dewey Avenue
Omaha, Nebraska

NEW JERSEY

Adolescent Clinic
Morristown Memorial Hospital
100 Madison Avenue
Morristown, New Jersey

NEW YORK: 1. NEW YORK CITY

Bronx

Adolescent Unit
The Bronx-Lebanon Medical Center
1650 Grand Concourse
Bronx, New York

The Division of Adolescent Medicine
Montefiore Hospital and Medical Center
111 East 210 Street
Bronx, New York

Brooklyn

Adolescent Unit
Jewish Hospital and Medical Center
Brooklyn, New York

Manhattan

Teenage Service
Beth Israel Hospital and Medical Center
10 Nathan Perlman Place
New York, New York

Teenage Clinic
Mt. Sinai School of Medicine
Fifth Avenue and 100 Street
New York, New York

Adolescent Clinic
New York University Medical Center
Bellevue Hospital
550 First Avenue
New York, New York

Adolescent Clinic
Roosevelt Hospital
459 West 59 Street
New York, New York

Adolescent Clinic
The New York Hospital
525 East 68 Street
New York, New York

2. *Long Island*

Adolescent Service
Long Island Jewish Hospital
270-05 76th Avenue
New Hyde Park, New York

3. *Rochester*

Adolescent Clinic
University of Rochester Medical Center
Rochester, New York

NORTH CAROLINA

Adolescent Clinic
Duke University Medical Center
Durham, North Carolina

NORTH DAKOTA

Adolescent Clinic
Quain and Ramstad Clinic
221 North Fifth Street
Bismarck, North Dakota

OHIO

Adolescent Clinic
General Hospital
Cincinnati, Ohio

Adolescent Health Services
Children's Hospital
561 South 17 Street
Columbus, Ohio

TEXAS

Adolescents' Division
Children's Medical Center
1935 Amelia Street
Dallas, Texas

VERMONT

Adolescent Clinic
Medical Center Hospital of Vermont
Burlington, Vermont

VIRGINIA

Adolescent Clinic
University of Virginia Hospital
Charlottesville, Virginia

Adolescent Clinic
Medical College of Virginia
Richmond, Virginia

WASHINGTON

Adolescent Clinic
University of Washington
4701-24th Avenue, N.E.
Seattle, Washington

Adolescent Clinic
Child Development and M. R. Center
University of Washington
Seattle, Washington

ABROAD

ARGENTINA

Municipal Center for Adolescents
Rawson Hospital
Buenos Aires, Argentina

AUSTRALIA

Princess Margaret Hospital for Children
Box D184, G.P.O.
Perth 6001, Western Australia

CANADA

Teen-Age Clinic
Montreal Children's Hospital
2300 Tupper Street
Montreal 25, Quebec, Canada

Adolescent Clinic
Ottawa Civic Hospital
Ottawa, Ontario, Canada

Adolescent Unit
Allan Memorial Institute
1025 Pine Avenue West
Montreal 2, Quebec, Canada

Adolescent Clinic
Hospital for Sick Children
555 University Avenue
Toronto 2, Ontario, Canada

FINLAND

Folkhalsan Teenage Clinic
Children's Hospital
Brandov 6, Helsinki, Finland

Birth Control Information

Planned Parenthood Regional Offices

ALABAMA

3030 Peachtree Road, N.W.
Atlanta, Georgia
(404) 233-3981

ALASKA

655 Sutter Street
San Francisco, California
(415) TU5-3120

ARIZONA

655 Sutter Street
San Francisco, California
(415) TU5-3120

ARKANSAS

4928 Burnet Road
Austin, Texas
(512) 452-6417

CALIFORNIA

655 Sutter Street
San Francisco, California
(415) TU5-3120

COLORADO

406 West 34 Street
Kansas City, Missouri
(816) JE1-2243

CONNECTICUT

515 Madison Avenue
New York, New York
(212) PL2-2257

DELAWARE

1605 Race Street
Philadelphia, Pennsylvania
(215) LO3--1731

DISTRICT OF COLUMBIA

1605 Race Street
Philadelphia, Pennsylvania
(215) LO3--1731

FLORIDA

3030 Peachtree Road, N.W.
Atlanta, Georgia
(404) 233-3981

GEORGIA

3030 Peachtree Road, N.W.
Atlanta, Georgia
(404) 233-3981

HAWAII

655 Sutter Street
San Francisco, California
(415) TU5-3120

IDAHO

655 Sutter Street
San Francisco, California
(415) TU5-3120

ILLINOIS

1111 East 54 Street
Indianapolis, Indiana
(317) 255-4126

INDIANA

1111 East 54 Street
Indianapolis, Indiana
(317) 255-4126

IOWA

406 West 34 Street
Kansas City, Missouri
(816) JE1-2243

KANSAS

406 West 34 Street
Kansas City, Missouri
(816) JE1-2243

KENTUCKY

1111 East 54 Street
Indianapolis, Indiana
(317) 255-4126

LOUISIANA

4928 Burnet Road
Austin, Texas
(512) 452-6417

MAINE

515 Madison Avenue
New York, New York
(212) PL2-2257

MARYLAND

1605 Race Street
Philadelphia, Pennsylvania
(215) LO3--1731

MASSACHUSETTS

515 Madison Avenue
New York, New York
(212) PL2-2257

MICHIGAN

1111 East 54 Street
Indianapolis, Indiana
(317) 255-4126

MINNESOTA

406 West 34 Street
Kansas City, Missouri
(816) JE1-2243

MISSISSIPPI

3030 Peachtree Road, N.W.
Atlanta, Georgia
(404) 233-3981

MISSOURI

406 West 34 Street
Kansas City, Missouri
(816) JE1-2243

MONTANA

406 West 34 Street
Kansas City, Missouri
(816) JE1-2243

NEBRASKA

406 West 34 Street
Kansas City, Missouri
(816) JE1-2243

NEVADA

655 Sutter Street
San Francisco, California
(415) TU5-3120

NEW HAMPSHIRE

515 Madison Avenue
New York, New York
(212) PL2-2257

NEW JERSEY

1605 Race Street
Philadelphia, Pennsylvania
(215) LO3-1731

NEW MEXICO

4928 Burnet Road
Austin, Texas
(512) 452-6417

NEW YORK

515 Madison Avenue
New York, New York
(212) PL2-2257

NORTH CAROLINA

3030 Peachtree Road, N.W.
Atlanta, Georgia
(404) 233-3981

NORTH DAKOTA

406 West 34 Street
Kansas City, Missouri
(816) JE1-2243

OHIO

1111 East 54 Street
Indianapolis, Indiana
(317) 255-4126

OKLAHOMA

4928 Burnet Road
Austin, Texas
(512) 452-6417

OREGON

655 Sutter Street
San Francisco, California
(415) TU5-3120

PENNSYLVANIA

1605 Race Street
Philadelphia, Pennsylvania
(215) LO3-1731

RHODE ISLAND

515 Madison Avenue
New York, New York
(212) PL2-2257

SOUTH CAROLINA

3030 Peachtree Road, N.W.
Atlanta, Georgia
(404) 233-3981

SOUTH DAKOTA

406 West 34 Street
Kansas City, Missouri
(816) JE1-2243

TENNESSEE

3030 Peachtree Road, N.W.
Atlanta, Georgia
(404) 233-3981

TEXAS

4928 Burnet Road
Austin, Texas
(512) 452-6417

UTAH

655 Sutter Street
San Francisco, California
(415) TU5-3120

VERMONT

515 Madison Avenue
New York, New York
(212) PL2-2257

VIRGINIA

3030 Peachtree Road, N.W.
Atlanta, Georgia
(404) 233-3981

WASHINGTON

655 Sutter Street
San Francisco, California
(415) TU5-3120

WEST VIRGINIA

3030 Peachtree Road, N.W.
Atlanta, Georgia
(404) 233-3981

WISCONSIN

1111 East 54 Street
Indianapolis, Indiana
(317) 255-4126

WYOMING

406 West 34 Street
Kansas City, Missouri
(816) JE1-2243

Suicide-Prevention Centers

Where to Call if You Need Some HELP (Adapted from the Bulletin of Suicidology of the National Institute of Mental Health)
(Open 24 hours a day, unless otherwise noted)

ALABAMA

Birmingham: (205) 323-7777
Decatur: (205) 355-8000
Florence: (205) 764-3431

ARIZONA

Phoenix: (602) 258-6301
Tucson: (602) 296-5411

CALIFORNIA

Bakersfield: (805) 325-1232
Berkeley: North County (415) 849-2212
South County (415) 537-1323
Ben Lomond: (408) 426-2342; (408) 688-1111
Carmel: (408) 373-0713
China Lake: (714) 446-5531
Davis: (916) 756-5000; (916) 756-5001
Fresno: (805) 485-1432
Garden Grove: (714) 636-2424; (213) 639-4673
Long Beach: (213) 435-7669
Los Angeles: (213) 620-0144; (213) 381-5111
(Operated by the Adolescent Unit of the Los Angeles Children's Hospital)

Napa and Solano Counties: (707) 643-2555 (Vallejo);
(707) 255-2555 (Napa); (707) 963-2555
(St. Helena); (707) 422-2555 (Fairfield)
Palm Springs: (714) 346-9502
Pasadena: (213) 798-0907; (213) 798-0908;
(213) 798-0909
Sacramento: (916) 454-5707; (916) 481-2233
San Anselmo: (415) 454-4524; (415) 454-4525
San Bernardino: (714) 886-4889
San Diego: (714) 239-0325 (10 a.m. to 12 p.m.,
Monday through Friday; 1 p.m. to 7 p.m.,
Saturday and Sunday)
San Francisco: (415) 558-4801 (weekdays)
(415) 221-1424
San Jose: (408) 287-2424
San Mateo: (415) 349-HOPE
Stockton: (209) 466-2961; (209) 466-2962
Ventura: (805) 648-2444
Walnut Creek: (415) 939-3232

COLORADO

Aurora: (303) 761-0620; (303) 364-9316
Colorado Springs: (303) 471-4357
Denver: (303) 394-8297; (303) 244-6835;
(303) 746-8485; (303) 757-0988; (303) 789-3073
Grand Junction: (303) 242-0577
Pueblo: (303) 544-1133

CONNECTICUT

Bridgeport: (203) 336-3876; (203) 366-3877

DELAWARE

Dover: (302) 678-1225
Lewes: (302) 856-6626
New Castle: (302) 656-4428

DISTRICT OF COLUMBIA

(202) 966-9511; (202) 966-9512 (weekdays);
(202) 629-5222

FLORIDA

Gainesville: (904) 376-4444
Jacksonville: (904) 384-6488
Miami: (305) 649-8206; (305) 649-8207;
  (305) 649-8208; (305) 379-2611
Orlando: (305) 241-3329
Rockledge: (305) 784-2433
St. Petersburg: (813) 347-0392
West Palm Beach and Boca Raton: (305) 848-8686
  (West Palm Beach); (305) 399-2244 (Boca Raton)

GEORGIA

Atlanta: (404) 572-2626

HAWAII

Honolulu: (808) 521-4555

ILLINOIS

Champaign: (217) 359-4141
Chicago: (312) 794-3609
East St. Louis: (618) 397-0963
Mt. Vernon: (618) 242-1511 (daytime);
  (618) 242-4600 (hospital switchboard night)
Peoria: (309) 691-7373; (309) 691-7374
Quincy: (217) 222-1166
Watseka: (815) 432-5111

INDIANA

Indianapolis: (317) 632-7575

IOWA

Keokuk: (319) 524-3873 (weekdays)

KANSAS

Garden City: (316) 276-7689
Kansas City: (913) 371-7171

Topeka: (913) 235-3434; (913) 235-3435
Wichita: (316) 268-8251 (business)

LOUISIANA

Baton Rouge: (504) 388-8222; (504) 388-1234

MAINE

Bangor: (207) 947-6143; 1-800-432-7810
 (WATS Toll Free Number)
Brunswick: (207) 443-3300
Portland: (207) 774-2767

MARYLAND

Baltimore: (301) 367-7800 (Ext. 8855)

MASSACHUSETTS

Boston: (617) 426-6600

MICHIGAN

Adrian: (313) 263-6737 (8 a.m. to 12 midnight,
 Monday through Thursday; 24 hours, Friday
 through Sunday)
Ann Arbor: (313) 761-9834; (313) 761-9835
Chelsea: (313) 475-2676
Detroit: (313) 875-5466
Flint: (313) 235-5677
Grand Haven: (616) 842-4357
Holland: (616) 396-4357; (616) 842-4357
Warren: (313) 758-6860
Ypsilanti: (616) 485-0440

MINNESOTA

Minneapolis: (612) 330-7777; (612) 330-7780
St. Paul: (612) 225-1515

MISSISSIPPI

Meridian: (601) 693-1001

MISSOURI

Kansas City: (816) 471-3000 (business)
St. Joseph: (816) 232-1655
St. Louis: (314) 868-6300

MONTANA

Browning: (406) 338-5525; (406) 226-4291
Great Falls: (406) 453-6511

NEBRASKA

Omaha: (402) 342-6290

NEVADA

Reno: (702) 323-6111

NEW HAMPSHIRE

Berlin: (603) 752-4431 (5½ days a week)

NEW JERSEY

Hammonton: (201) 561-1234
Metuchen: (201) 549-6000
Plainfield: (201) 561-4800

NEW MEXICO

Las Cruces: (505) 524-9241

NEW YORK

Brooklyn: (212) 462-3322

Buffalo: (716) 854-1966
East Meadow: (516) 538-3111
Ithaca: (607) 272-1616
New York: (212) 686-3061; (212) 736-6191
Niagara Falls: (716) 285-3515
Rochester: (716) 275-4445
White Plains: (914) 949-0121

NORTH CAROLINA

Durham: (919) 688-5504
Gastonia: (704) 867-6373
Greensboro: (919) 275-2852
Jacksonville: (919) 346-6292
Roanoke Rapids: (919) 537-2909
Sanford: (919) 776-5431

NORTH DAKOTA

Bismarck: (701) 255-4124
Fargo: (701) 232-4357
Grand Forks: (701) 772-7268
Minot: (701) 838-5555

OHIO

Akron: (216) 434-9144
Ashtabula: (216) 993-6111
Athens: (614) 592-3917
Canton: (216) 452-9811
Columbus: (614) 221-5445; (614) 221-5451
Dayton: (513) 223-4777
Kent: (216) 672-4357; (216) 672-4358 (12 hours
    a day, Monday through Thursday; 24 hours a day,
    Friday through Sunday)
Newark: (614) 344-1111 (8 p.m. to 2 p.m., Monday
    through Thursday; noon Friday to 6 a.m. Sunday)
Toledo: (419) 478-0361
Zanesville: (614) 452-8403

OREGON

Corvallis: (503) 752-7030

PENNSYLVANIA

Bethlehem: (215) 691-0660
Philadelphia: (215) 686-4420

SOUTH CAROLINA

Greenville: (803) 239-1021

TENNESSEE

Knoxville: (615) 637-9711
Memphis: (901) 274-7473 (dial CRISIS-3);
 (901) 525-1717
Nashville: (615) 244-7444

TEXAS

Abilene: (915) 673-3132
Amarillo: (806) 376-4251; (806) 376-4442
Corpus Christi: (512) 883-6244; (512) 883-6245
Dallas: (214) 521-5531
Fort Worth: (817) 336-3355
San Antonio: (512) 734-5726: (512) 735-8328
Wichita Falls: (817) 723-0821; (817) 823-0822

UTAH

Salt Lake City: (801) 484-8761

VIRGINIA

Portsmouth: (703) 399-6393

WASHINGTON

Bremerton: (206) 373-2402
Olympia: (206) 357-3681
Seattle: (206) 325-5550
Spokane: (509) 838-4428; (509) 838-4429;
 (509) 838-4430

WEST VIRGINIA

    Charleston: (304) 346-3332
    Huntington: (304) 523-3448

WISCONSIN

    Eau Claire: (715) 834-5522
    Elkhorn: (414) 245-5011
    Madison: (608) 251-2345
    Milwaukee: (414) 258-2040 (Ext. 3143)

A Guide To Information
For Narcotics Addicts

(Field Offices for the Narcotic Addict Rehabilitation
Branches of the National Institute of Mental Health)

ALABAMA

1783 Washington Avenue
Atlanta, Georgia
(404) 526-7574

ALASKA

11000 Wilshire Boulevard
Los Angeles, California
(213) 824-7456

ARIZONA

11000 Wilshire Boulevard
Los Angeles, California
(213) 824-7456

ARKANSAS

106 Broadway
San Antonio, Texas
(512) 225-5511

CALIFORNIA

11000 Wilshire Boulevard
Los Angeles, California
(213) 824-7456

COLORADO

11000 Wilshire Boulevard
Los Angeles, California
(213) 824-7456

CONNECTICUT

26 Federal Plaza
New York, New York
(212) 264-1041

DELAWARE

26 Federal Plaza
New York, New York
(212) 264-1041

DISTRICT OF COLUMBIA

5454 Wisconsin Avenue
Chevy Chase, Maryland
(301) 496-7277

FLORIDA

1783 Washington Avenue
Atlanta, Georgia
(404) 526-7574

GEORGIA

1783 Washington Avenue
Atlanta, Georgia
(404) 526-7574

HAWAII

11000 Wilshire Boulevard
Los Angeles, California
(213) 824-7456

IDAHO

11000 Wilshire Boulevard
Los Angeles, California
(213) 824-7456

ILLINOIS

127 North Dearborn Street
Chicago, Illinois
(312) 353-4205

INDIANA

127 North Dearborn Street
Chicago, Illinois
(312) 353-4205

IOWA

127 North Dearborn Street
Chicago, Illinois
(312) 353-4205

KANSAS

127 North Dearborn Street
Chicago, Illinois
(312) 353-4205

KENTUCKY

5454 Wisconsin Avenue
Chevy Chase, Maryland
(301) 496-7277

LOUISIANA

106 Broadway
San Antonio, Texas
(512) 225-5511

MAINE

26 Federal Plaza
New York, New York
(212) 264-1041

MARYLAND

5454 Wisconsin Avenue
Chevy Chase, Maryland
(301) 496-7277

MASSACHUSETTS

26 Federal Plaza
New York, New York
(212) 264-1041

MICHIGAN

127 North Dearborn Street
Chicago, Illinois
(312) 353-4205

MINNESOTA

127 North Dearborn Street
Chicago, Illinois
(312) 353-4205

MISSISSIPPI

1783 Washington Avenue
Atlanta, Georgia
(404) 526-7574

MISSOURI

127 North Dearborn Street
Chicago, Illinois
(312) 353-4205

MONTANA

11000 Wilshire Boulevard
Los Angeles, California
(213) 824-7456

NEBRASKA

127 North Dearborn Street
Chicago, Illinois
(312) 353-4205

NEVADA

11000 Wilshire Boulevard
Los Angeles, California
(213) 824-7456

NEW HAMPSHIRE

26 Federal Plaza
New York, New York
(212) 264-1041

NEW JERSEY

26 Federal Plaza
New York, New York
(212) 264-1041

NEW MEXICO

11000 Wilshire Boulevard
Los Angeles, California
(213) 824-7456

NEW YORK

26 Federal Plaza
New York, New York
(212) 264-1041

NORTH CAROLINA

5454 Wisconsin Avenue
Chevy Chase, Maryland
(301) 496-7277

NORTH DAKOTA

127 North Dearborn Street
Chicago, Illinois
(312) 353-4205

OHIO

127 North Dearborn Street
Chicago, Illinois
(312) 353-4205

OKLAHOMA

106 Broadway
San Antonio, Texas
(512) 225-5511

OREGON

11000 Wilshire Boulevard
Los Angeles, California
(213) 824-7456

PENNSYLVANIA

26 Federal Plaza
New York, New York
(212) 264-1041

RHODE ISLAND

26 Federal Plaza
New York, New York
(212) 264-1041

SOUTH CAROLINA

1783 Washington Avenue
Atlanta, Georgia
(404) 526-7574

SOUTH DAKOTA

127 North Dearborn Street
Chicago, Illinois
(312) 353-4205

TENNESSEE

1783 Washington Avenue
Atlanta, Georgia
(404) 526-7574

TEXAS

106 Broadway
San Antonio, Texas
(512) 225-5511

UTAH

11000 Wilshire Boulevard
Los Angeles, California
(213) 824-7456

VERMONT

26 Federal Plaza
New York, New York
(212) 264-1041

VIRGINIA

5454 Wisconsin Avenue
Chevy Chase, Maryland
(301) 496-7277

WASHINGTON

11000 Wilshire Boulevard
Los Angeles, California
(213) 824-7456

WEST VIRGINIA

5454 Wisconsin Avenue
Chevy Chase, Maryland
(301) 496-7277

WISCONSIN

127 North Dearborn Street
Chicago, Illinois
(312) 353-4205

WYOMING

11000 Wilshire Boulevard
Los Angeles, California
(213) 824-7456

PUERTO RICO

5454 Wisconsin Avenue
Chevy Chase, Maryland
(301) 496-7277

VIRGIN ISLANDS

5454 Wisconsin Avenue
Chevy Chase, Maryland
(301) 496-7277

A Glossary of Drug-Related Terms

Acid: LSD, LSD-25 (lysergic acid diethylamide)
Acidhead: Frequent user of LSD

Bag: Packet of drugs
Bang: Injection of drugs
Barbs: Barbiturates
Bennies: Benzedrine (form of amphetamine)
Bindle: Packet of narcotics
Blank: Extremely low-grade narcotics
Blast: Strong effect from a drug
Blow: Inhale (usually heroin)
Blue angels: Amytal, a barbiturate
Blue velvet: Paregoric (camphorated tincture of opium) and Pyribenzamine (an antihistamine) mixed and injected
Bombita: Amphetamine injection, sometimes taken with heroin
Bread: Money
Bum trip: Bad experience with psychedelics
Busted: Arrested
Button: Head of peyote cactus

Cap: Container in which heroin is dissolved; part of the "works"; or: a capsule
Chippie: The desire for a drug in the absence of addiction
Chipping: Taking narcotics occasionally
Christmas trees: Tuinals (amobarbitol and secobarbitol)
CIBA: Doriden (glutethamide), a form of depressant
Coasting: Under the influence of drugs
Coke: Cocaine
Cokie: Cocaine addict

Cold turkey: Sudden withdrawal from a drug, usually heroin, without medication (from the resultant goose-flesh, which resembles the skin of a cold plucked turkey)

Coming down: The end of a spree on drugs

Connection: A pusher, i.e, a drug supplier

Cop: To obtain heroin

Cop out: To quit, take off, confess, defect, inform

Crashing: The end of an amphetamine binge

Crash pad: Place where the user withdraws from amphetamines

Crystals: LSD or methedrine

Cubehead: Frequent user of LSD

Cut: Dilute drugs by adding milk sugar or another inert substance

Dealer: A pusher, i.e., a drug supplier

Deck: A $10 packet of drugs (usually heroin)

Dexies: Dexedrine (form of amphetamine)

DET: A synthetic hallucinogen

Deuce: A $2 packet of drugs (usually heroin)

Dime bag: A $10 packet of drugs (heroin or marijuana)

Dirty: Possessing drugs, liable to arrest if searched

DMT: A synthetic hallucinogen

Dollies: Dolophines (methadone)

DOM: STP (a synthetic hallucinogen)

Dope: Heroin (a decade ago was used for airplane glue)

Doper: Person who uses drugs regularly

Downs: Sedatives (barbiturates, Doriden, tranquilizers)

Drop: To ingest a drug

Dummy: Purchase which did not contain narcotics

Dynamite: High-grade heroin

Fix: Injection of narcotics

Flash: The immediate effect of injecting a drug; a "rush"

Flip: Become psychotic

Floating: Under the influence of drugs

Freak out: To lose contact with reality through drugs (usually hallucinogens)

Fuzz: The police

Gage: Marijuana

Good trip: Happy experience with psychedelics
Goofballs: Barbiturates (sleeping pills)
Grass: Marijuana

H: Heroin
Hard stuff: Heroin
Hash: Hashish
Hay: Marijuana
Head: A chronic user of drugs (usually LSD or marijuana)
Hearts: Dexedrine (because of the shape)
Heat: The police
High: Under the influence of drugs
Holding: Having drugs in one's possession
Hooked: Addicted
Hophead: Narcotics addict
Horse: Heroin
Hustle: To steal, beg, or prostitute oneself for money for drugs
Hype: Narcotics addict

Joint: Marijuana cigarette
Jolly beans: Pep pills (amphetamines)
Jones: A habit (usually heroin)
Joy-pop: Inject narcotics irregularly
Junkie: Drug user (usually heroin)

Kick: To stop a habit; to withdraw

LSD: D-lysergic acid diethylamide (synthetic hallucinogen)
Layout: Equipment for injecting drug (works)
Lemonade: Poor heroin

M: Morphine
Main: To inject drugs intravenously
Mainline: Same as Main
(The) Man: The police
Manicure: Remove the dirt, seeds, and stems from marijuana
Mary Jane: Marijuana
Mesc: Mescaline, the alkaloid in peyote
Meth: Methamphetamine, methedrine (an amphetamine), speed

Mikes: Micrograms (millionths of a gram)

Narc: Narcotics detective
Nickel bag: A $5 packet of drugs (usually heroin or marijuana)
Nod: To doze off while on heroin

O.D.: Overdose of drugs (heroin or barbiturates)

Panic: Shortage of narcotics on the market
Pillhead: Heavy user of pills, barbiturates or amphetamines or both
Pop: Inject drugs
Pot: Marijuana
Pothead: Heavy marijuana user
Pusher: Drug peddler

Quill: A matchbook cover for sniffing Methedrine, cocaine, or heroin

Rainbow: Tuinal, because of its red and blue capsule (a barbiturate)
Red devil: Seconal (a barbiturate)
Reefer: Marijuana cigarette
Reentry: Return from trip
Roach: Marijuana cigarette butt
Roach holder: Device for holding the butt of a marijuana cigarette
Run: A binge on amphetamines
Rush: The immediate effect of injecting a drug (usually heroin)

Satch cotton: Cotton used to strain drugs before injection; may be used again if supplies are gone
Scag: Heroin
Score: To buy drugs
Shoot up: To inject drugs intravenously
Shooting gallery: Place where addicts inject
Skin-pop: To inject drugs beneath the skin
Smack: Heroin
Smoke: Wood alcohol
Sniff: To inhale airplane glue or cleaning fluid; never used to refer to heroin inhalation

Snort: To inhale heroin

Snow: Cocaine

Speed: Methedrine (when injected intravenously)

Speedball: An injection of a stimulant and a depressant, originally heroin and cocaine

Speedfreak: Habitual user of speed

Spike: Needle, broken eyedropper, or other sharp object used to inject drugs

STP: A synthetic hallucinogen

Stash: Supply of drugs in a secure place

Stick: Marijuana cigarette

Stoolie: Informer

Strung out: Addicted (to heroin)

Tea: Marijuana

Tooies: Tuinal (a barbiturate)

Tracks: Scars along veins after many injections

Tray: A $3 packet of drugs (usually heroin)

Trip: Experience while on hallucinogens

Tripping out: High on psychedelics

Turned on: To be exhilarated (usually with reference to hallucinogens)

Turps: Elixir of Terpin Hydrate with codeine, a cough syrup

25: LSD (from its original designation, LSD-25)

Ups: Stimulants, amphetamines, cocaine

Weed: Marijuana

Works: Equipment used for preparing an injection of drugs

Yellow jacket: Nembutal (a barbiturate)

Yen sleep: A drowsy, restless state during the withdrawal period

INDEX

A

Abscesses, 105. *See also* specific locations

Abdominal injuries, 142

Abdominal pain, 62-63. *See also* specific disorders

Abortion, 58, 76, 82-83

Acne, 126-29, 133, 135-36

Adrenal glands, 50, 126, 186

Alcohol, 107, 155

Amenorrhea, 55, 56-59, 124

Amphetamines, 58, 151, 174-77, 178; for menstrual cramps, 60

Amytal, 178

Androgens (male hormones), 125. *See also* Hormones; specific disorders

Anemia, 104-05, 109-10

Anorexia nervosa, 28, 48-51

Anus, 52 *(see also* Rectum); itching, 66

Aortic stenosis, 140

Appendicitis, 63, 86

Areolas, 16, 126

Arm injuries, 143, 144

Arthritis, 87, 104

Aspiration pneumonia, 159

Asthma, 94-97, 160

Athletics, 139-44

Atropine, 60, 171-72

Axillary hair (underarm hair), 18, 20, 26

B

Back *(See also* Spinal curvature)*: fractured, 143; round, 121-22

Barbiturates, 94-95, 102, 151, 178-79

Baseball, 144

Basilar artery migraine, 101-02

Bath dermatitis, 129-30

Beards (and beardlessness), 19, 20, 22, 128

Bed-wetting, 147-49

Biological revolution, 186-87

Birth control, 75-81 *(See also* Oral contraceptives); information services on, 203-06

Birth defects. *See* Pregnancy

Blackheads, 127, 129

D

E

T

Do you really know who you are?

Do you know how you look to others? Do you know all about yourself—even the things you don't want to admit? Do you realize that you could be wrecking your chances for happiness and fulfillment without ever suspecting it?

BE THE PERSON YOU WERE MEANT TO BE offers a dramatically effective new way of taking a good honest look at yourself—and making the changes you want to become a whole new you.

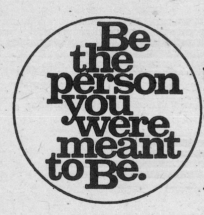

by Dr. Jerry Greenwald

A DELL BOOK $1.75

If you enjoyed I'M OK—YOU'RE OK, you will want to read this great book that sold over a quarter of a million copies in hardcover.

Love and Will

by ROLLO MAY

* *over 4 months on the bestseller lists*
* *a selection of 6 book clubs*
* *winner of the Ralph Waldo Emerson Award*

"An extraordinary book on sex and civilization . . . An important contribution to contemporary morality."

—*Newsweek*

". . . a rich and useful book, one that deserves a thoughtful audience."

—*Saturday Review*

A DELL BOOK $1.75
Also available in a Delta edition $2.95